Patanjali Yoga Sutras and their Interpretations

Patanjali Yoga Sutras and their Interpretations

Dr. Rajendra Singh

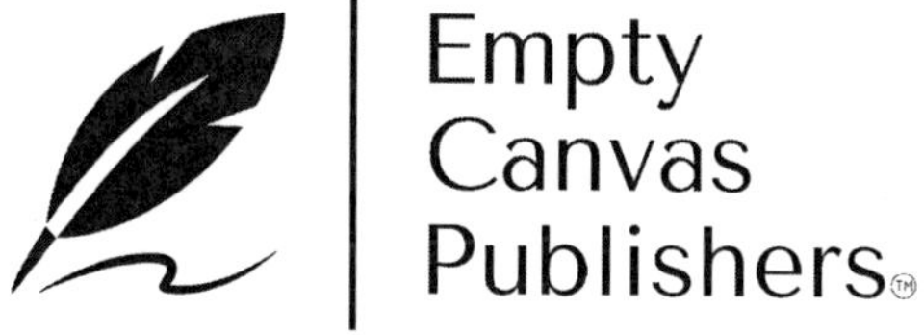

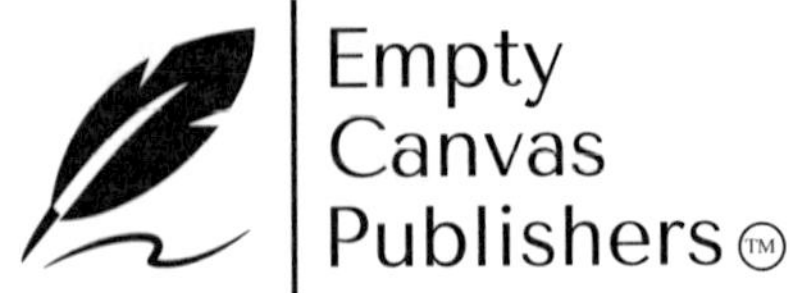

Corporate Office:
EMPTY CANVAS PUBLISHERS™
4435-36/7, 1st Floor
Ansari Road, Daryaganj
New Delhi-110002
Email: emptycanvaspublishers@gmail.com

Registered Office:
EMPTY CANVAS PUBLISHERS™
AP-119C, Pitam Pura
New Delhi-110034 (India)
www.emptycanvaspublishers.com

Edition : 2022

ISBN: 978-81-949219-9-8

Patanjali Yoga Sutras and Their Interpretation

Author: Dr. Rajandra Singh

Author takes full ownership of the literal content of the book and is solely responsible for ensuring that his work doesn't hurt religious and political sentiments of people.

Published by:
EMPTY CANVAS PUBLISHERS™
New Delhi-110034 (India)

Processed And Printed in India

Preface

This book is an attempt at an English translation of Patanjali's Yogasutra with commentary rendered in current psychological idiom. It features an extensive Introduction to the context and attempts to draw out conclusions on the implications of yoga theory and practices to current psychological knowledge.

The name Patanjali means "falling from joined hands" (in Sanskrit, the word patat means falling and anjali means joined hands). As with most great Indian mystics, sages and priests, there are mythical stories explaining their incarnation (or reincarnation). The myth widely held for Patanjali is that he deeply desired to share with the world the teachings of Yoga and other knowledge so he chose to be reborn as a seven-year old boy, falling from the ethereal world directly into his mother's hands, a Brahmin woman named Gonika. For this reason she named him Patanjali (from David Gordon White's book, The Yoga Sutra of Patanjali: A Biography).

Although no one is certain, scholars believe Patanjali lived sometime between 500 BCE and 200 CE. Patanjali is not only credited with writing the Yoga Sutras, but also works on Ayurveda and Sanskrit grammar. Because of his prolificacy, some scholars question whether Patanjali was one person or if the name refers to a collective group of sages and teachers. Where everyone is in agreement though is that Patanjali brilliantly codified the vast oral tradition of Yoga into a concise written form. He did not develop Yoga, the science existed thousands of years before Patanjali.

Yoga is a group of ancient spiritual practices originating in India. As a general term in Hinduism it has been defined as referring to "technologies or disciplines of asceticism and meditation which are thought to lead to spiritual experience and profound understanding or insight into the nature of existence." Yoga is also intimately connected to the religious beliefs and practices of the other Indian religions. Outside India, Yoga is mostly associated with the practice of Asanas (postures) of Hatha Yoga or as a form of exercise, although it has influenced the entire Indian religions family and other spiritual practices throughout the world.

Hindu texts discussing different aspects of yoga include the Upanishads, the Bhagavad Gita, the Yoga Sutras of Patanjali, the Hatha Yoga Pradipika, the Shiva Samhita, and many others. Major branches of Yoga include: Hatha Yoga, Karma Yoga, Jnana Yoga, Bhakti Yoga, and Raja Yoga. Raja Yoga, known simply as Yoga in the context of Hindu philosophy, is one of the six orthodox (astika) schools of thought, established by the Yoga Sutras of Patanjali.

This is a reference book. All the matter is just compiled and edited in nature, taken from the various sources which are in public domain.

This book thus provides the psychological context and the relevance of studies of yoga for advancing the existing psychological knowledge. Yoga psychology provides the foundation for Indian psychology, an emerging discipline, rooted in classical Indian tradition.

—*Editor*

Contents

CHAPTER

1

Introduction

The tradition of Patañjali in the oral and textual tradition of the Yoga Sûtras is accepted by traditional Vedic schools as the authoritative source on Yoga, and it retains this status in Hinducircles into the present day. In contrast to its modern Western transplanted forms, Yoga essentially consists of meditative practices culminating in attaining a state of consciousness free from all modes of active or discursive thought, and of eventually attaining a state where consciousness is unaware of any object external to itself, that is, is only aware of its own nature as consciousness unmixed with any other object. This state is not only desirable in its own right, but its attainment guarantees the practitioner freedom from every kind of material pain or suffering, and, indeed, is the primary classical means of attaining liberation from the cycle of birth and death in the Indic soteriological traditions, that is, in the theological study of salvation in India. The Yoga Sûtras were thus seen by all schools, not only as the orthodox manual for guidance in the techniques and practices of meditation, but also for the classical Indian position on the nature and function of mind and consciousness, for the mechanisms of action in the world and consequent rebirth, and for the metaphysical underpinnings and description of the attainment of mystical powers.

In terms of literary sources, there is evidence as early as the oldest Vedic text, the Rg Veda (c. 1200 - c. 1500 B.C.E.), that there were yogi-like ascetics on the margins of the Vedic world. In terms of the archaeological record, seals found in

Indus Valley sites (c. 3000 - c. 1500 B.C.E.) with representations of figures seated in a clear yogic posture (the most famous figure is seated inpadmasana, lotus pose, with arms extended and resting on the knees in a classical meditative posture), suggest that, irrespective of its literary origins, Yoga has been practiced on the Indian subcontinent for well over 4000 years. However, it is in the late Vedic age, marked by the fertile speculations expressed in a genre of texts called the Upanisads (c. 800 - c. 600 B.C.E.), that practices that can be clearly related to classical Yoga are first articulated in literary sources.

While the Upanisads are especially concerned with jñ na, or understanding Brahman, the Absolute Truth, through the cultivation of knowledge, there are also several unmistakable references to a technique for realising Brahman (in its localised aspect of atman) called Yoga. As with the Upanisads in general, we do not find a systematic philosophy here, but mystico-poetic utterances, albeit profound in content. The Mahâbhârata Epic, which is the largest literary epic in the world, also preserves significant material representing the evolution of Yoga, indeed, the term "yoga" and "yogî" occur about 900 times throughout the Epic.

Usually dated somewhere between the 9th–4th centuries C.E., the Epic exhibits the transition between the origins of Yoga in the Upanisadic period and its expression in the systematised traditions of Yoga as represented in the classical period by Patañjali. Nestled in the middle of the Epic, the well-known Bhagavad Gîtâ (c. 4th century B.C.E.), devotes a good portion of its bulk to the practices of Yoga, which it considers to be "ancient".

This, of course, indicates that practices associated with Yoga had gained wide currency in the centuries prior to the common era, with a clearly identifiable set of basic techniques and generic practices, and we will here simply allude to the fact that scholars have long pointed out a commonality of vocabulary, and concepts between the Yoga Sûtras (YS) and Buddhist texts. All this underscores the fact that there was a cluster of numerous interconnected and cross-fertilizing variants of meditational Yoga - Buddhist and Jain as well as Hindu - prior to Patañjali, all drawn from a common but variegated pool of terminologies, practices and concepts (and, indeed, many strains continue to the present day). Of closer relevance to the Sûtras is the fact that the history of Yoga is inextricable from that of the Sâmkhya tradition. Samkhya provides the metaphysical infrastructure for Yoga, and thus is indispensable to an understanding of Yoga. While both Yoga and Sâmkhya share the same metaphysics and the common goal of liberating purusa from its encapsulation, their methods differ.

Sâmkhya occupies itself with the path of reasoning to attain liberation, specifically concerning itself with the analysis of the manifold ingredients of prakrti from which the purusa was to be extricated, and Yoga more with the path of meditation, focusing its attention on the nature of mind and consciousness, and the techniques of concentration in order to provide a practical method through which the purusa can be isolated and extricated. Sâmkhya seems to have been perhaps the earliest philosophical system to have taken shape in the late Vedic period, and has permeated almost all subsequent Hindu traditions; indeed the classical Yoga of Patañjali has been seen as a type of neo-Sâmkhya, updating the old Sâmkhya tradition to bring it into conversation with the more technical philosophical traditions that had emerged by the 3–5th centuries C.E., particularly Buddhist thought. In fact, Sâmkhya and Yoga should not be considered different schools until a very late date: the first reference to Yoga itself as a distinct school seems to be in the writings of Sankara in the 9th century C.E. Yoga and Sâmkhya in the Upanisads and Epic simply refer to the two distinct paths of salvation by meditation and salvation by knowledge, respectively.

One might add, as an aside, that from the 900-odd references to Yoga in the Mahâbhârata, there are only two mentions of asana, posture, the third limb of Patañjali's system.

Neither the Upanisads nor the Gîtâ mention posture in the sense of stretching exercises and bodily poses (the term is used as "seat" rather than bodily postures), and Patañjali himself only dedicates three brief sutras from his text to this aspect of the practice.

The reconfiguring, presentation and perception of Yoga as primarily or even exclusively asana in the sense of bodily poses, then, is essentially a modern Western phenomenon and finds no precedent in the premodern Yoga tradition. From this rich and fertile post-Vedic context, then, emerged an individual called Patañjali whose systematisation of the heterogeneous practices of Yoga came to be authoritative for all subsequent practitioners and his system eventually reified into one of the six schools of classical Indian philosophy. It is important to stress here that Patañjali is not the founder or inventor of Yoga, the origins of which, as noted above, had long preceded him in primordial and mythic times. Patañjali systematised the pre-existing traditions and authored what came to be the seminal text for Yoga discipline. There was never one uniform school of Yoga, or Ur-Yoga (or of any Indic school of thought for that matter): there was a plurality of variants, and certainly different conceptualisations of meditative practices that were termed Yoga.

For example, while Patañjali organises his system into eight limbs, and the Mahâbhârata, too, speaks of Yoga as having eight "qualities", as early as in the Maitrî Upanisad of the 2nd century B.C.E., there is reference to a six-limbed Yoga, as there is in the Visnu Purâna. Along similar lines, there are various references to the twelve yogas and seven dharanas found in the Epic Mahâbhârata. Yoga is thus best understood as a cluster of techniques, some more and some less systematised, that pervaded the landscape of ancient India. These overlapped and were incorporated into the various traditions of the day such as the jñana, knowledge-based traditions, providing these systems with a practical method and technique for attaining an experienced-based transformation of consciousness. Patañjali's particular systematisation of these techniques was in time to emerge as the most dominant, but by no means exclusive, version.

Indeed, internal to his own text, in his very first sutra, atha yoga anusasanam, Patañjali indicates that he is continuing the teachings of Yoga (the verbal prefix anu indicates the continuation of the action denoted by the verb), and the traditional commentators certainly perceive him in this light. In point of fact, the tradition itself ascribes the actual origins of Yoga to the legendary figure Hiranyagarbha. Moreover, evidence that Patañjali was addressing an audience already familiar with the tenets of Yoga can be deduced from the Yoga Sûtras themselves. For example, on occasion, Patañjali will mention one member of a list of items followed by "etc.,", thereby assuming his audience to be familiar with the remainder of the list. But, in short, because he produced the first systematised treatise on the subject, Patañjali was to become the prime or seminal figure for the Yoga tradition after his times, and was accepted as such by other schools. To all intents and purposes, his Yoga Sûtras were to become the canon for the mechanics of generic Yoga, so to speak, that other systems tinkered with, and flavoured with their own theological trappings.

As with the reputed founders of the other schools of thought, very little is known about Patañjali himself. Tradition, first evidenced in the commentary of Bhoja Râja in the 11th century C.E., considers him to be the same Patañjali who wrote the primary commentary on the famous grammar by PâG ini, and also ascribes to him authorship of a treatise on medicine. There is an ongoing discussion amongst scholars as to whether this was likely or not, but there is not much to be gained by challenging the evidence of traditional accounts in the absence of alternative evidence to the contrary that is uncontroversial or at least adequately compelling.

Patañjali's date can only be inferred from the content of the text itself. Unfortunately, as with most classical Sanskrit texts from the ancient period, early Sanskrit texts tend to be impossible to date with accuracy, and there are always dissenters against whatever dates become standard in academic circles. Most scholars seem to date the text shortly after the turn of the common era, (c. 1st - c. 2nd century C.E.), but it has been placed as early as several centuries before the common era. Other than the fact that the text does not postdate the 5th century C.E., the date of the Yoga Sûtras cannot be determined with exactitude.

The Sûtra writing style is that used by the philosophical schools of ancient India (thus we have Vedânta Sûtras, Nyâya Sûtras, etc.). The term "sûtra," (from the Sanskrit root su, cognate with "sew") literally means a thread, and essentially refers to a terse and pithy philosophical statement in which the maximum amount of information is packed into the minimum amount of words. Knowledge systems were handed down orally in ancient India, and thus source material was kept minimal partly with a view to facilitating memorisation.

Being composed for oral transmission and memorisation, the Yoga Sûtras, and sûtra traditions in general, allowed the student to "thread together" in memory the key ingredients of the more extensive body of material with which the student would become thoroughly acquainted. Thus, each sûtra served as a mnemonic device to structure the teachings and facilitate memorisation, almost like a bullet point that would then be elaborated upon.

This very succinctness - the Yoga Sûtras contain about 1200 words in 195 sûtras - and the fact that the sûtras are in places cryptic, esoteric and incomprehensible in their own terms points to the fact that they served as manuals to be used in conjunction with a teacher. Therefore, it is an unrealistic (if not impossible) task to attempt to bypass commentary in the hope of retrieving some original pure, pre-commentarial set of Ur-interpretations

Knowledge systems in ancient Indian were transmitted orally, from master to disciple, with an enormous emphasis on fidelity towards the original set of Sûtras upon which the system is founded, the master unpacking the dense and truncated aphorisms to the students. Periodically, teachers of particular prominence wrote commentaries on the primary texts of many of these knowledge systems. Some of these gained wide currency to the point that the primary text was always studied in conjunction with a commentary, particularly since texts such as the Yoga Sûtras were designed to be unpacked because they contain numerous sûtras that are incomprehensible without further elaboration. One cannot overstress, therefore, that our understanding of Patañjali's text is completely dependent on the interpretations of later commentators: it is incomprehensible, in places, in its own terms.

In terms of the overall accuracy of the commentaries there is an a priori likelihood that the interpretations of the Sutras were faithfully preserved and transmitted orally through the few generations from Patañjali until the first commentary by Vyâsa in the 5th Century C.E. Certainly, the commentators from Vyâsa onwards are remarkably consistent in their interpretations of the essential metaphysics of the system for over fifteen hundred years, which is in marked contrast with the radical differences in essential metaphysical understanding distinguishing commentators of the Vedânta school (a Râmânuja or a Madhva from a Sankara, for example).

While the 15thcentury commentator Vijñânabhiksu, for example, may not infrequently quibble with the 9thcentury commentator Vâcaspati Miúra, the differences generally are in detail, not essential metaphysical elements. And while Vijñânabhiksu may inject a good deal of Vedântic concepts into the basic dualism of the Yoga system, this is generally an addition (conspicuous and identifiable) to the system rather than a reinterpretation of it. There is thus a remarkably consistent body of knowledge associated with the Yoga school for the best part of a millennium and a half, and consequently one can speak of "the traditional understanding" of the

Sûtras in the premodern period without overly generalising or essentialising.

The first extant commentary by the legendary Vyâsa, typically dated to around the 4-5th century C.E., was to attain a status almost as canonical as the primary text by Patañjali himself. Consequently, the study of the Yoga Sûtras has always been embedded in the commentary that tradition attributes to this greatest of literary figures. Practically speaking, when we speak of the philosophy of Patañjali, what we really mean (or should mean) is the understanding of Patañjali according to Vyâsa: it is Vyâsa who determined what Patañjali's abstruse Sûtras meant, and all subsequent commentators elaborated on Vyâsa. The Vyâsa Bhâsya (commentary) becomes inseparable from the Sûtras; an extension of it. From one sutra of a few words, Vyâsa might write several lines of comment without which the sutra remains incomprehensible. Vyâsa's commentary, the Bhâsya, thus attains the status of canon, and is almost never questioned by any subsequent commentator. Subsequent commentators base their commentaries on unpacking Vyâsa's Bhâsya - rarely critiquing it, but rather expanding or elaborating upon it. It is this point of reference that produces a marked uniformity in the interpretation of the Sûtras in the pre-modern period. The next commentary is called the Vivarana, attributed to the great Vedântin Sankara in the 8th - 9th century C.E. It has remained unresolved since it was first questioned in 1927 whether the commentary on the Yoga Sûtras assigned to Sankara is authentically penned by him. The next best known commentator is Vâcaspati Misra, whose commentary, the Tattvavai Sâradî, can be dated with more security to the 9th century C.E. Vâcaspati Miúra was a prolific intellectual, penning important commentaries on the Vedânta, Sâmkhya, Nyâya and Mîmâmsâ schools in addition to his commentary on the Yoga Sûtras, and was noteworthy for his ability to present each tradition in its own terms, without displaying any overt personal predilection.

A fascinating Arabic translation of Patañjali's Sûtras was undertaken by the famous Arab traveler and historian al-Bîrunî (973–1050 C.E.), the manuscript of which was discovered in Istanbul in the 1920's. Roughly contemporaneous with al-Bîrunî is the 11th century King Bhoja, poet, scholar and patron of the arts, sciences and esoteric traditions, in whose commentary, called the Râjamârtanð"a, there are on occasion very valuable insights to be found. In the 15th century, Vijñânabhiksu wrote a most insightful and useful commentary after that of Vyâsa's, the Yogavârttika. Vijñânabhiksu was another prolific scholar, noteworthy for his attempt to harmonise Vedânta and Sâmkhya concepts.

In the 16th century C.E., another Vedântin, Râmânanda Sarasvatî, wrote his commentary, called Yogamaniprabhâ, which also adds little to the previous commentaries. But there are valuable insights contained in the Bhâsvatî by Hariharânanda Âranya, written in Bengali, from a context nearer our own times, a standpoint exposed to Western thought, but still thoroughly grounded in tradition. While many other commentaries have been written, these are the primary commentaries written in the pre-modern era. The commentaries written in the modern period, many of which have made massive adjustments to modernity or the sensitivities of the Western market, are beyond the scope of this discussion, which limits itself to classical Yoga philosophy.

The Yoga Sûtras is divided into four padas, chapters. The first, samadhi pada, defines Yoga as the complete cessation of all active states of mind, and outlines various stages of insight that stem from this. The chapter points to the ultimate goal of Yoga, which is content-less awareness, beyond even the most supreme stages of insight.

The second, sadhana pada, outlines the various practices, and moral and ethical observances that are preliminary requirements to serious meditative practice. The third, vibhk ti pada, primarily deals with various super-normal powers that can accrue to the practitioner when the mind is in extreme states of concentration. There seems to have been a widespread culture in ancient India of engaging in Yoga-like practices but not in pursuit of the real goal of Yoga as defined by Patañjali, but rather in quest of such super-normal powers; this chapter can be read as Patañjali's warning against being side-tracked in this way. The fourth, kaivalya pada deals with liberation, and, amongst other things, contains Patañjali's response to the Buddhist challenge.

HISTORY OF YOGA

Indus Valley Seals: Several seals discovered at Indus Valley Civilization (c. 3300-1700 BC) sites depict figures in a yoga or meditation like posture. The most widely known of these was named the "Pashupati seal" by its discoverer, John Marshall, who believed that it represented a "proto-Shiva" figure. Many modern authorities discount the idea that this "Pashupati" (Lord of Animals, Sanskrit pashupati) represents a Shiva or Rudra figure.

There is considerable evidence to support the idea that the image's posture "is a form of ritual discipline, suggesting a precursor to yoga" according to archaeologist Gregory Possehl (who also questions the proto-Shiva theory).

He points to sixteen other specific "yogi glyptics" in the corpus of Mature Harappan artifacts as pointing to Harappan devotion to "ritual discipline and concentration". These images show that the yoga pose "may have been used by deities and humans alike". He suggests that yoga goes back to the Indus Valley Civilization.

Gavin Flood characterizes these views as "speculative", saying that it is not clear from the 'Pashupati' seal that the figure is seated in a yoga posture, or even that the shape is intended to represent a human figure, though it is nevertheless possible that there are echoes of Shaiva iconographic themes, such as half-moon shapes resembling the horns of a bull. Other authorities do support the idea that the 'Pashupati' figure shows a figure in a yoga or meditation posture. They include Archaeologist Jonathan Mark Kenoyer, current Co-director of the Harappa Archaeological Research Project in Pakistan and Indologist Heinrich Zimmer.

In 2007, terracota seals were discovered in the Cholistan Desert in Pakistan. Punjab University Archaeology Department Chairman Dr. Farzand Masih described one of the seals as similar to the previously discovered Mohenjodaro seals, with three pictographs on one side and a "yogi" on the other side.]

Literary Sources

Ascetic practices (tapas) are referenced in the Brahmanas (900 BC and 500 BC), early commentaries on the vedas. In the Upanishads, an early reference to meditation is made in Brihadaranyaka Upanishad, one of the earliest Upanishads (approx. 900 BC). The main textual sources for the evolving concept of Yoga are the middle Upanishads, (ca. 400 BC), the Mahabharata (5th c. BC) including the Bhagavad Gita (ca. 200 BC), and the Yoga Sutras of Patanjali (200 BCE-300 CE).

Bhagavad Gita

The Bhagavad Gita ('Song of the Lord'), thought to have been composed in roughly the 2nd century BC, uses the term yoga extensively in a variety of senses. Of many possible meanings given to the term in the Gita, most emphasis is given to these three:

- Karma yoga: The yoga of action
- Bhakti yoga: The yoga of devotion
- Jnana yoga: The yoga of knowledge

The influential commentator Madhusudana Sarasvati (b. circa 1490) divided the Gita's eighteen chapters into three sections, each of six chapters. According to his method of division the first six chapters deal with Karma yoga, the middle six deal with Bhakti yoga, and the last six deal with Jnana (knowledge). This interpretation has been adopted by some later commentators and rejected by others.

PATANJALI YOGA SUTRAS

Samadhi Pada

The famous definitional aphorism: *"Yogas chitta-vritti-nirodhah – yoga is the control of thought waves in the mind"* (1.2). The chapter deals with the absolute true consciousness or Isvara and describes the problems an individual soul is likely to face in its quest for merger with the Divine Soul. It begins with an analyses of human thought processes or vrittis, which deter us from realising our true selves.

The Samadhi Pada advises the restraint of such natural inclinations of the mind and discusses the problems encountered while trying to harness it. Then it elucidates the concept of Isvara, the supreme consciousness and the various gradations of samadhi which is a self-absorbed, detached state of being. Here again, the possible mental distractions are stated and the best methods of conquering these impediments are discussed.

The central doctrine of Yoga philosophy is that nothing exists beyond the mind and its consciousness, which is the only ultimate reality. The objective of this philosophy is to uproot misconceptions about the existence of external 'realities' from the minds of men. It believes that it is possible to reach this stage of self realisation through regular practice of certain yogic meditative processes that bring a complete withdrawal or detachment from all false sources of knowledge and inculcates an inner sense of balanced calm and tranquility. It may be observed from the above narration that the focal point of the Yoga Sutras is the human mind and its examination.

Classification of the Mind

While the first three stages are negative and cause impediments to the healthy growth of the mind, the latter two are the desired states of mind conducive to meditation. Various yogic practices such as certain yogasanas, pranayama, dhyana, dharana and samadhi are designed for achieving the absolute balanced state of mind.

When the mind is in its earliest stage of disturbance, it lacks judgment and is generally hyperactive, unable to ignore external stimuli. The next stage of the stupefied state of mind is distinguished by inertia, lethargy, sluggishness, vice, ignorance and sleep. The state of distracted mind is an advanced stage of the disturbed mind, when it still lacks consistency and is unable to quieten down. One-pointed and balanced states of mind are the mental levels at which, the mind almost ceases to be affected by the turbulence of mortal existence. They are the calmest and most peaceful states of mind. This tranquil state of mind is the nearest to the inner stillness one can ever get. This state of mind is highly conducive for concentration and meditation, which is why the yoga system lays emphasis on various yogic meditational practices.

Under the conditions of the one-pointed state of mind, one attains to the state of perfect concentration where there is a clear cognition of the object. The last stage of balanced mind is that rare state of being, where the mind is totally undisturbed and purified by the flow of positive energy. It is the ultimate desired mental stage in yogic practices. It is at this immaculate state alone that one is able to realise the true nature of the soul. In this state of mind there is a total suppression of all modifications leading to Samadhi, where no object is recognised and the Purusha remains established in His own intrinsic state. Then he becomes a Mukta, a liberated soul, freed from all the bondages of nature (prakriti).

Modifications of the Mind

The inner instruments of thought process (antahkarana) consist of Chitta, the mind-stuff (a store-house or memory), mind (manas) and intellect (buddhi). The waves of thoughts, feelings and emotions that arise in it due to the impact of the sense-objects upon it through the five sense-organs like the eyes, ears etc., are called modifications of the mind (chittavrittis). All our thoughts, emotions and psychological states fall within any one of these sections. These five again are further subdivided into two mental types: *viz.,* malevolent and benevolent where the first type causes afflictions while the second one does not create any trouble. Misapprehension, conceptualization and deep sleep are considered to be the three main causes of various afflictions while the categories of comprehension and memory are viewed more positively which are conducive to meditation and the attainment of kaivalya or detachment from the material world.

Misapprehension is equivalent to ignorance (avidya) in Yoga philosophy. And knowledge borne out of misconceptions such as mistaking a rope for a snake and vice versa are false, leading to afflictions of the greatest kind. Conceptualization is also considered to be a source of ignorance because it is the comprehension of an object based only on words and expressions, even though the object is absent *e.g.,*beliefs such as the existence of horned rabbits or son of a barren woman. Although such ideas can be conceived they are all erroneous knowledge which does not correspond with anything in existence. Deep sleep is also thought to be a negative modification of the mind.

During this mental state the mind is overcome with heaviness and no other activities are present. This state is virtually a withdrawal from the external world, when one is left without any control over one's consciousness. It may be noted that the dream state and the waking state are not modifications because while dreaming, our minds are occupied with conceptualization and while awake, the mind is concerned with the categories of comprehension or misapprehension. Memory is concerned with the recalling of stored impressions, or rather the mental retention of conscious experiences. The one-pointed and absolutely balanced states of mind are free from these categories of modifications while in the other three states they are present.

PRE PATANJALI PERIOD

The historical evidences of yoga were seen up to 4500 B.C. So the time before 4500 B.C. and after 4500 B.C. up to Patanjali period is considered as pre Patanjali period. The main sources which we can get during those times are Vedas, Upanishads, Smrti, Teaching of Buddha, Jainism, Panini, Epics and Puranas.

Vedas

Among the available Vedas four are important, namely Rigveda, Yajurveda, Samaveda and Atharvaveda. There is no any direct explanation of word yoga in Vedas, whereas the word 'dhira', is mentioned in all Vedas. The meaning of dhira is self-realised.

The sitting posture *i.e.*, Asana, the Pranayama, the Mudras, Meditation techniques, the cleanliness Yama and Niyama, the Dharanas are explained in Vedas. The asanas explained in Vedas are mainly for the purpose of meditation. The sun salutation was the part of routine activity during that time. The Pranayama that is told in the Yajurveda, which is practiced during the regular practice, is same as Anuloma Viloma. The various types of meditation techniques are also explained in the Vedas. The practice of mudras is also explained in the Vedas. The Vedas also explain about the Tapas, Vratas and the ultimate aim of them are to attain Moksa (liberation).

Upanishads

Upanishads are the essences of the Vedas. Among the available Upanishads, 10 are important. The important Upanishads that have explanations about yoga are as follows. The Panchakosha theory is explained in Taittariya Upanishad is the main theory used in the treatment of diseases through yoga. Kathopanishad explains procedure to attain Samadhi. This Upanishad explains the qualities of soul. The Kenopanishad, the Ishavasya Upanishad, Shwetasvatara Upanishads are also gives details about yoga.

Smṛti

The Smrits are the texts, which deal about the disciplines that one has to follow in his life. The main smrtis, which give details about yoga, are Manusmrti, Yajnavalkya Smrti, and Harita Smriti.

According to the smrtis there are four stages in life, they are:

- Brahmacarya
- Grhastha
- Vanaprastha
- Sanyasa

The Smrtis also give details about the lifestyles that we have to follow during these different stages of life. According to smrtis one has to sit in a seat that is prepared from Darbha (one type of grass) for meditation. The asanas good for meditation are also explained in smrtis.

Jainism

In Jainism also yoga is explained. According to Jainism the movement of the mind and body towards the soul is called yoga.

Teachings of Buddha

According to Buddha body is a fit vehicle to get the tranquility of mind. For getting the steadiness of mind the body should become steady at first. The methods of meditation are also explained in teachings of Buddha. According to that there are two types of meditations, Suksma dhyana and Nirhara dhyana.

Panini: He was a famous grammarian of Sanskrit. He wrote 8 chapters lessons of grammar, Astadhyayi. The usage of word yoga is there in his work.

The Epics: The Ramayana and Mahabharata are the two main epics that give the details about yoga. Ramayana consists of 24,000 slokas distributed among seven chapters. The great book of yoga known asYoga Vasistha was written in this time. In Ramayana the moral disciplines, Yama and Niyama are explained in detail. We can see the definition for Dharma in this book. Mahabharata is another important epic, which gives details about yoga. The Bhagavad-Gita is known as jewel of Mahabharata gives the definition for yoga.

Puranas: Among the available puranas eighteen are important. Out of these few puranas give details about yoga. The Bhagavata purana explains Bhakti yoga. Linga Purana gives the details about Yama, Niyama and Pranayama. Vayu Purana gives details about Pratyahara, Dharana, and Dhyana.

Patanajali Period [500 BC - 800BC]

The period between 500 BC and 800 AD is considered as Patanjali's period. Patanjali systematised yoga in the form of sutras. Patanjlai was the author of classics in three important fields. He wrote a treatise on grammar; the Mahabbhasya. He has also written book on Ayurveda. He has the credit of compiling Yoga sutra.

Patanjali's yoga sutra consists of 196 sutras, it is divided into four chapters, and they are:

- *Samadhi Pada:* This chapter deals with the nature of Samadhi.
- *Sadhana Pada:* This chapter deals with the methods for refining the body mind and senses.
- *Vibhuti Pada:* In this chapter the properties of Yoga and art of integration through concentration, meditation and absorption. The manifestation of super natural power is discussed.
- *Kaivalya Pada:* In this final section, Patanjali draws the attention of the Yogi to the soul. The various types of Samadhi are explained in this chapter.

These Yoga sutras explain every aspects of yoga in systematically.

Post Patanjali Period

The time after Patanjali up to today is known as post Patanjali Period. The yoga developed gradually after the period of Patanjali. Many classical texts about yoga were written during these periods. The great personalities of yoga and their texts on yoga are as follows. *Shankaracharya (8th Century): Sri Shankaracharya proposed Advaita Philosophy. He has written Yoga Taravali, which tells about Hatha Yoga and Saundarya lahari that explains Kundalini Yoga. He has also written commentary on Patanjala Yoga Sutras. Ramanujacarya (11th Century): He has written the book Tantra Sara that explains Kundalini yoga. He proposed Vishistadvaita philosophy.

PSYCHOLOGICAL GROWTH AND YOGA

Four Stages of Life

Each stage should ideally last twenty five years, as normal life span is thought to be 100 years for "highly developed" individuals.

All four stages must be passed in order to receive self-realisation:

- *Student:* Occupational skills, as well as character development through emotional and spiritual discipline are the focus of this stage. The goal is to become a mature, productive individual, fully equipped to live a harmonious and productive life.
- *Householder:* Carrying on a family business and raising a family are the focus of this stage in life.

The householder seeks satisfaction in family pleasures, vocational success, and in being an active responsible citizen of the community.

- *Forest Dweller:* Refers to the gradual retirement from family and occupation. The husband and wife may move to a smaller house in the woods, or may withdraw in large part from social and community affairs. They are still available to their children to give advise and counsel.
- *Renunciant:* Entrance to this stage is marked by a ritual which resembles funeral rites. The individual gives up

all responsibilities and social obligations and is now free to pursue self-realisation without external demands or restrictions.

Five Obstacles to Self-Realisation within Yoga

- *Ignorance:* The major obstacle to growth. The basis for all suffering is ignorance of our true identity. An ignorant person is someone who concentrates all their conscious energy on the outside world, instead of focusing on the one true source of joy, the self.
- *Egoism:* Results when we identify the Self with the body. Identification with the body leads to fear, desire, and limitation.
- *Desire and Aversion:* The longing for pleasure and the recoiling from pain. These afflictions tie an individual to the external world. A major aim of Yoga is to overcome our sensitivity to pain, pleasure, success, and failure. The Yogic principle of non-attachment is to enjoy what one has, but not to desire what one is missing.
- *Fear:* Fear is the constant terror of death, and stems from body identification, rather than Self identification.

Other Aspects of Psychology within Yoga

- *The Body:* Depending upon which branch of Yoga you are indoctrinated in, the body can be seen as a positive source for spiritual growth, or as an onerous source of desire, fear, and aversion which prevents one from self-realisation.
- *Social Relationships:* Your social relationships vary, depending upon your level of self-realisation. Before realisation, our social relationships are due to the socio-cultural traditions of our upbringing. After realisation we can act within society, but we are not of society.

"Learn to see God in all persons You will know what divine love is when you begin to feel your oneness with every human being, and not before that time" (Yogananda, 1986)

Willpower

Principles of austerity and denying one's desires through fasting, yogic positions, and celibacy is a long lasting tradition of Hinduism and Yoga.

- *Tapas:* the tradition of practicing austerity and restraint, to show self-control over one's own bodily desires.
- Exercise of will also provides Yoga students with the direct experience of confronting laziness, low self-discipline, and similar non-desirable personality traits.
- *Emotions:* Yoga distinguishes between painful waves and non-painful waves of consciousness.

Painful waves are thoughts and emotions which increase ignorance, confusion, or attachment.

They do not have to be unpleasant (*i.e.* pride), but they do further distance you from realisation of the self.

Non-painful waves of love, generosity, and courage should be cultivated to create positive subconscious tendencies, which will lead to positive karmic actions. However, Even positive emotional states are transcended by someone who has reached self-realisation.

Intellectual Development in the Yogic Tradition

Intellect is the increased understanding through personal experience. Yogics who attempt to study the Veda without putting into practice the words of the verses are practicing a sterile intellectualism which will not lead to realisation.

Personal Reflection is necessary to grow the intellect. Meditation, Fasting, Silence, and austere living are all methods to help aid in the self-analysis of personal reflection.

Conclusions of Yoga and Modern Personality

Many Parallels exist between this ancient religious philosophy and modern theories of personalities.

The Freudian structure of consciousness, and the idea that the desires of the ID are hidden from usual awareness seems to have much in common with the body-spirit division within Hinduism. In Yoga, you try to realise the self. In psychotherapy you try to uncover those repressed memories of the unconscious. Jung's stages of life seem to closely resemble the Yogic stages of life in many details. Jung's descriptions of Extraversion and Introversion as turning inward or outward of psychic energy resembles the two thrusts of consciousness within Yoga.

Adler's, Roger's and Maslow's descriptions of personality and how to treat people seems to have some Hindu flavour as well. Think of the roles the guru must take, and then think about the relationship to the Adlerian ideas of Social interest, and the treatment philosophy of all three that congruence, empathy, and understanding are crucial for psychological growth within a therapeutic setting. The special relationship between the guru and his disciple, and the modeling the guru does for the disciple is analogous to the modern therapist-client relationship with Client Centered treatment philosophies. Maslow's goal of Self-Actualisation seem to flow from the Yogic concepts of self-realisation. Maslow's conception of B-values seems closely related to the Karma-Yoga (Yoga of Action) philosophy.

FEATURED ON YOGA

Patanjali's Yoga Sutras outline a path for obtaining divine oneness, self-realisation or, as Nicolai Bachman says, in his book The Path of the Yoga Sutras, a deep understanding of the core of who you are. Among yogis and spiritual seekers, this promise is very inviting. What is even more attractive is that the path is laid out in 195 short verses (or 196, depending on the school of thought). You could easily read the entire Yoga Sutras in 30 minutes or less. However, making sense of these pithy lines is a different, and much longer, story. Like yoga, studying the Sutras could span a lifetime.

There are dozens of translations of Patanjali's Yoga Sutras, and they vary because the terse verses leave much room for interpretation.

The name Patanjali means "falling from joined hands" (in Sanskrit, the word patat means falling and anjali means joined hands). As with most great Indian mystics, sages and priests, there are mythical stories explaining their incarnation (or reincarnation). The myth widely held for Patanjali is that he deeply desired to share with the world the teachings of Yoga and other knowledge so he chose to be reborn as a seven-year old boy, falling from the ethereal world directly into his mother's hands, a Brahmin woman named Gonika. For this reason she named him Patanjali (from David Gordon White's book, The Yoga Sutra of Patanjali: A Biography).

Although no one is certain, scholars believe Patanjali lived sometime between 500 BCE and 200 CE. Patanjali is not only credited with writing the Yoga Sutras, but also works on Ayurveda and Sanskrit grammar. Because of his prolificacy, some scholars question whether Patanjali was one person or if the name refers to a collective group of sages and teachers. Where everyone is in agreement though is that Patanjali brilliantly codified the vast oral tradition of Yoga into a concise written form. He did not develop Yoga, the science existed thousands of years before Patanjali. In India, the ancient tradition of orally transmitting knowledge through the chanting of mnemonic verses is still practiced today, helping students recall knowledge passed down from their teachers.

In Sanskrit, the word sutra means thread, and each densely packed and succinctly written Sutra represents a large amount of knowledge. Chanting the verses helps students with memorisation and pronunciation. The belief is that students are not ready to question their understanding of a teaching until they have committed the knowledge to memory and have mastered the pronunciation.

The inspiration of the Yoga Sutras comes from the Vedas, which are the most ancient preserved texts in India, as well as the foundation of Hindu spirituality. Today, Patanjali's Yoga Sutras remain the primary text on Yoga philosophy. The first verse of the Yoga Sutras is translated as: "Now the teachings of yoga." Today, a reader may assume that Patanjali's Yoga Sutras are about asanas, or postures, which is the modern day connotation of Yoga. Although, after reading just a few lines, it is clear that Patanjali is concerned with meditation and ultimately, Self-Realisation. The text says very little about asana. What is shared about asana relates to finding a comfortable sitting position for meditation.

Patanjali's Yoga Sutras are divided into four chapters, or Padas: 1). Meditative Absorption, 2). Practice, 3). Mystic Powers and 4). Absolute Independence. The Sutras explain the nature of reality, our misunderstanding of the nature of reality and the practices necessary to see reality clearly. As Chip Hartranft says in his book, The Yoga-Sutra of Patanjali, "Though brief, the Yoga Sutras manage to cut to the heart of the human dilemma."

The main problem, Patanjali says, is a misunderstanding about Consciousness and Pure Awareness. They are separate, but are often perceived by humans to be one and the same.

Patanjali's solution for this is to allow Consciousness to settle from the whirling thoughts, sensations and emotions to a point where it can reflect Pure Awareness back to itself. This is addressed right away, in the second verse: Yoga is to still the patterning of consciousness.

When this is achieved, we connect with our source of true happiness - Pure Awareness. The path Patanjali lays out is a journey within, accessible to anyone, offering deep, universal insight that guides practitioners to freedom.

Today, the philosophy from the Sutras that yoga practitioners are most familiar with is The Eightfold Path, or Ashtanga Yoga (unrelated to the asana system founded by

Pattabhi Jois), which appears in Chapter 2, Verses 28 - 32. Ancient lore says that when a student approached a teacher to study Yoga, the teacher would require him to master the Yamas and Niyamas, the first two limbs of the Eightfold Path, before returning to learn asana.

In brief, the Yamas and Niyamas are ethical principles and the foundation of Yogic thought.

The Yamas, which mean 'restraints' in Sanskrit, include:

- Ahimsa: non-violence
- Satya: truthfulness
- Asteya: non-stealing
- Bramacharya: non-excess (often also translated as abstinence)
- Aparigraha: non-possessiveness

The Yamas are a guide to having a right relationship with the world. As humans, we are part of a greater whole, and every action we make has a corresponding reaction.

When practiced and embraced, the Yamas allow us to live in the world in a harmonious and peaceful way with all people, creatures and the environment, contributing to the health and happiness of society.

The Niyamas, which means 'observances' in Sanskrit, include:

- Saucha: purity
- Santosha: contentment
- Tapas: self-discipline
- Svadyaya: self-study
- Ishvara Pranidhana: surrender.

These observances guide our relationship with self and how to live meaningfully and soulfully. One of the most beautiful, and accessible, translations of the Yamas and Niyamas can be found in Donna Farhi's book: Yoga Mind, Body and Spirit: A Return to Wholeness. Volumes have been written on just the Yamas and Niyamas, and like the Sutras, can be a life-long practice and study.

Following the Yamas and Niyamas on the Eight-Limbed Path, are Asana, Pranayama (breath control), Pratyahara (withdrawal of the senses), Dharana (concentration), Dhyana (meditation) and Samadhi (a state of ecstasy). Like Ayurveda, Yoga's sister science, Yoga was given to humanity as a gift. Ayurvedic philosophy is focused on longevity and leading a life of well-being. In the case of Yoga, the practices are dedicated to ending the 'mundane' cycle of birth, death and rebirth. Ultimately, Patanjali's Yoga Sutras speaks to the greatest desire of every human being - how to end the cause of suffering and find eternal happiness.

TANTRA

Tantra, also called Tantrism and Tantric religion, is an Asian tradition of beliefs and meditation and ritual practices that seeks to channel the divine energy of the macrocosm or godhead into the human microcosm, in order to attain siddhis and moksha. It arose in India no later than the 5th century CE, and had a strong influence on both Hinduism and Buddhism. The term "tantrism" or "tantricism" is an anglicism derived from "tantra", used since the 19th century to refer to a complex and broad body of non-Vedic teachings.

Tantrism

According to André Padoux, "Tantrism" is a western term and notion, and not a category which is being used by the so-called "Tantrists" themselves. The term was introduced by 19th century Indologists who thought that the Tantras were only a very limited aspect of Indian culture. Yet, accoridng to Padoux, "[Tantra was] so pervasive that it was not regarded as being a distinct system."

Robert Brown also notes that the term "tantrism" is a construct of Western scholarship, not a concept from the religious system itself. *Tântrikas* (practitioners of Tantra) did not attempt to define Tantra as a whole; instead, the Tantric dimension of each South Asian religion had its own name:

- Tantric Shaivism was known to its practitioners as the *Mantramârga.*
- Shaktism is practically synonymous and parallel with Tantra, known to its native practitioners as "Kula marga" or "Kaula".
- Tantric Buddhism has the indigenous name of the Vajrayana.
- Tantric Vaishnavism was known as the Pancharatra.

Tantrika

According to Padoux, the term "tantrika" is based on a comment by Kulluka Bhatta, who made a distinction between *vaidika* and *tantrika* forms of revelation. These coincide with two different approaches to ultimate reality, namely a Vedic-Brahmanical approach, and approaches based on other texts.

Tantra

Tantra Sanskrit: often simply means "treatise" or "exposition". Literally it can be said to mean "loom, warp, weave"; hence "principle, continuum, system, doctrine, theory", from the verbal root *tan* "stretch, extend, expand", and the suffix *tra* "instrument".

The *Kâmikâ-tantra* gives the following explanation of the term *tantra*:

- Because it elaborates (*tan*) copious and profound matters, especially relating to the principles of reality (*tattva*) and sacred mantras, and because it provides liberation (*tra*), it is called a *tantra*.

The 10th-century Tantric scholar RâmakaGm ha, who belonged to the dualist school Úaiva Siddhânta, gives another definition:

- A tantra is a divinely revealed body of teachings, explaining what is necessary and what is a hindrance in the practice of the worship of God; and also describing the specialized initiation and purification ceremonies that are the necessary prerequisites of Tantric practice.

Scholarly Definitions

According to David N. Lorenzen, two different kind of definitions of Tantra exist, a "narrow definition" and a "broad definition." According to the narrow definition, Tantrism, or "Tantric religion," refers only to the traditions which are based on the Tantras, Samhitas and Agamas. This definition refers primarily to a tradition which is primarily based in the higher social classes, which were literate, and lived in or close by urban centers.

According to the broad definition, Tantra refers to a broad range of religious traditions with a "magical" orientation. This includes the upper class texts and traditions, but also practices and rituals from lower social classes, which were less educated, and lived more in the rural areas.

According to David Gordon White, Tantra is that Asian body of beliefs and practices which, working from the principle that the universe we experience is nothing other than the concrete manifestation of the divine energy of the godhead that creates and maintains that universe, seeks to ritually appropriate and channel that energy, within the human microcosm, in creative and emancipatory ways.

Components

David N. Lorenzen gives the following components of the broadly defined Tantric religion which can be documented:

1. "Shamanic and yogic beliefs and practices;"
2. "Sakta worship, especially worship of the Matrkas and demon-killing forms of Hindu and Buddhist goddesses;"
3. "Specific schools of Tantric religion such as the Kapalikas and Kaulas;"
4. "The Tantric texts themselves."

Characteristics

André Padoux notes that there is no consensus among scholars which elements are characteristic for Tantra, nor is there any text which contains all those elements. And most of those elments can also be found in non-Tantric traditions. According to Anthony Tribe, a scholar of Buddhist Tantra, Tantra has the following defining features:

1. Centrality of ritual, especially the worship of deities
2. Centrality of mantras
3. Visualisation of and identification with a deity
4. Need for initiation, esotericism and secrecy
5. Importance of a teacher (guru, *âcârya*)
6. Ritual use of mandalas (*maG ala*)
7. Transgressive or antinomian acts
8. Revaluation of the body
9. Revaluation of the status and role of women
10. Analogical thinking (including microcosmic or macrocosmic correlation)
11. Revaluation of negative mental states

History

Origins

According to Brian K. Smith "all [...] attempts at locating the temporal and cultural origins of Tantrism remain theoretical and speculative." According to Andre Padoux, "the history of Tantrism is impossible to write." Although some elements of Tantra may be quite ancient, Hindu Tantrism as a related complex of religious rituals and practices probably originated ca. 500-600 CE.

Pre-Vedic

Some elements of Tantra may be quite ancient. Some scholars postulate pre-Vedic origins of Tantra. According to Bhattacharya, Tantric elements can be discerned in the Zhob and Kulli cultures of Baluchistan at the 4th millennium BCE. Terracotta figurines may be the earliest tokens of the Mother Goddess. These cultures, in their late phase, overlapped with the Harappan culture of the Indus Valley, which may have preserved these proto-Tantric elements. In contrast, the early vedic religion did not support this kind of Mother Goddess worship, and likewise didn't support the Yogic elements of the pre-Vedic north-Indian culture. Nevertheless, a synthesis emerged in which proto-Tantric elements found a place in the Vedic culture. Likewise, Manoranjan Basu postulates pre-Vedic origins of Tantra in the pre-Vedic culture of north-India, including the Indus Valley Civilization. The confrontation between the two cultures resulted in a synthesis in which proto-Tantric elements survived.

Worship of Female Deities

According to Lorenzen, the worship of female deities has a long history in India. Despite its patriarchal character, some Vedic hymns are dedicated to female deities.

Other Vedic texts, such as the *Mahabharata*, also contain references to the cruel manifestations of the Mother Goddess, especially Mahishamardini, who is identified with Durga-Parvati. The earliest depictions of Mahishamardini date from the 6th century CE, indicating the development of the Shakti-worship.

Goddess-worship became more tantric with the rise of the seven Matrikas, which are mentioned in the '*Mahabharata* and the early Puranic literature. They are also mentioned in the stone inscription of Visvavarman, which is dated at 423CE, and often regarded oldest written evidence of Tantrism. Another important mention of the Matrikas is in the *Markandeya Purana*, an early text of the Shakti worship.

Tantric Movement

Hindu Tantrism as a related complex of religious rituals and practices probably originated ca. 500-600 CE. Stone inscriptions make clear that Tantric deities were already worshipped in the 5th century, and Tantra may have been well established by the 6th or 7th century, by the end of the Gupta period.

Tantric Sects

The earliest reliable references to the Kapalikas are in Hâla's Gatha-saptasati (3rd-5th century CE) and in two texts written by Varâhamihira (c. 500–575 CE). In the 7th century CE more references to the Kapalikas appear. Epigraphic references to the Kaulas are rare. Reference is made in the early 9th century to *vama* (left-hand) Tantras of the Kaulas.

Tantras

The Hindu Tantras cannot be attested before 800 CE. According to Flood, the earliest date for the Tantras is 600 CE, though most of them were composed from the 8th century onward. By the 10th century an extensive corpus existed. According to Flood, the main areas for the composition of the tantras were Kashmir and Nepal. The Tantric traditions regard the Tantras, also called agamas, to be superior to the Vedas. While the vedic orthodoxy rejected the Tantras, the Tantric followers incorporated the Vedic revelations within their own systems, as revelations of a lower level.

According to Flood, the Tantras probably arose among non-Brahmanical ascetics who lived at the cremation grounds. They were representants of an ascetic ideal which lived among people of lower social classes. By the early medieaval times, their practices included the imitation of the gods they worshipped, which they appeased with various gifts such as non-vegetarian food, alcohol and sexual substances. They invited their deities to possess them, meanwhile keeping control and thereby gaining power. These ascetics were supported by low castes living at the cremation places.

Spread of Tantra

Tantrism flourished between the 8th or 9th century and the 14th century. This was a period of great social and economical change in India, which saw the rise of feudalism, and the start of the Muslim era. After the end of the Gupta Empire and the collapse of the Harsha Empire, power was decentralised in India. Several larger kingdoms emerged, with "countless vassal states". The kingdoms were ruled by a feudal system, with smaller kingdoms dependent on protection from larger ones. "The great king was remote, was exalted and deified." This was reflected in the Tantric mandala, which could depict the king at its centre.

The disintegration of central power led to religious regionalism and rivalry. Local cults and languages developed, and the influence of "Brahmanic ritualistic Hinduism" diminished. Rural devotional movements arose with Shaivism, Vaisnavism, Bhakti and Tantra, although "sectarian groupings were only at the beginning of their development." Religious movements competed for recognition from local lords. Buddhism lost its stature, and began to disappear from India.

By the tenth or eleventh century Tntra had spread all over India. Tantric movements led to the formation of a number of Hindu and Buddhist esoteric schools, also infuencing the Jain religious tradition. According to Flood, Tantrism has been so pervasive that all of Hinduism after the eleventh century, perhaps witht he exception of the vedic Srauta tradition, is influenced by it. All forms of Saiva, Vaisnava and Smarta religion, even those forms which wanted to distance themselves from Tantrism, absorbed elements derived from the Tantras.

Tantrism further spread with the silk road transmission of Buddhism to East and Southeast Asia, and also influenced the Bön tradition of Tibet.

Goal

Tantric ritual seeks to access the supra-mundane through the mundane, identifying the microcosm with the macrocosm. The Tantric aim is to sublimate (rather than negate) reality. The Tantric practitioner seeks to use *prana* (energy flowing through the universe, including one's body) to attain goals which may be spiritual, material or both.

Tantric teachings are passed on orally in a teacher-student relationship. Initiation by a teacher is necessary for the practice to be successful.

Practices

Rituals are the main focus of the *Tantras*. Rather than one coherent system, Tantra is an accumulation of practices and ideas. Because of the wide range of communities covered by the term, it is problematic to describe tantric practices definitively.

Sadhanas

A number of techniques (sadhana) are used as aids for meditation and achieving spiritual power:

- Dakshina: Donation or gift to one's teacher
- Diksha: Initiation ritual in which one receives shaktipat
- Yoga, including breathing techniques (*pranayama*) and postures (*asana*), is employed to balance the energies in the body/mind.
- Mudras, or hand gestures
- Mantras: reciting syllables, words, and phrases
- Singing of hymns of praise (*stava*)
- Mandalas
- Yantras: symbolic diagrams of forces at work in the universe
- Visualization of deities and Identification with deities
- Puja (worship ritual)
- Animal sacrifice
- Use of taboo substances such as alcohol, cannabis, meat and other entheogens.
- Prayashcitta - an expiation ritual performed if a puja has been performed wrongly
- Nyasa
- Ritual purification (of idols, of one's body, etc.)
- Guru bhakti (devotion) and puja

- Yatra: pilgrimage, processions
- Vrata: vows, sometimes to do ascetic practices like fasting
- The acquisition and use of siddhis or supernomal powers. Associated with the left hand path tantra.
- Ganachakra: A ritual feast during which a sacramental meal is offered.
- Ritual Music and Dance.
- Maithuna: ritual sexual union (visualized or with an actual physical consort).
- Dream yoga

Mandalas

According to David Gordon White, mandalas are a key element of Tantra. They represent the constant flow and interaction of both divine, demonic, human and animal energy or impulses (*kleshas, cetanâ, tanhâ*) in the universe. The mandala is a mesocosm, which mediates between the "transcendent-yet-immanent" macrocosm and the microcosm of mundane human experience. The godhead is at the center of the mandala, while all other beings, including the practitioner, are located at various distances from this center. Mandalas also reflected the medieaval feudal system, with the king at its centre. The godhead is both transcendent and immanent, and the world is regarded as real, and not as an illusion. The goal is not to transcend the world, but to realize that the world is the manifestation of the godhead, while the "I" is "the supreme egoity of the godhead." The world is to be seen with the eyes of the godhead, realizing that it is a manifestation as oneself. The totality of all that is a "realm of Dharma" which shares a common principle. The supreme is manifest in everyone, which is to be realized through Tantric practice.

MANTRA, YANTRA, NYASA

The words *mantram, tantram* and *yantram* are rooted linguistically and phonologically in ancient Indian traditions.

Mantram denotes the chant, or "knowledge." *Tantram* denotes philosophy, or ritual actions. *Yantram* denotes the means by which a person is expected to lead their life.

The mantra and yantra are instruments to invoke higher qualities, often associated with specific Hindu deities such as Shiva, Shakti, or Kali. Similarly, *puja* may involve focusing on a *yantra* or *mandala* associated with a deity.

Each mantra is associated with a specific Nyasa. Nyasa involves touching various parts of the body at specific parts of the mantra, thought to invoke the deity in the body. There are several types of Nyasas; the most important are *Kara Nyasa* and *Anga Nyasa*.

Identification with Deities

Visualisation

The deities are internalised as attributes of *Ishta devata* meditations, with practitioners visualizing themselves as the deity or experiencing the *darshan* (vision) of the deity. During meditation the initiate identifies with any of the Hindu gods and goddesses, visualising and internalising them in a process similar to sexual courtship and consummation. The *Tantrika* practitioner may use visualizations of deities, identifying with a deity to the degree that the aspirant "becomes" the *Ishta-deva* (or meditational deity).

Classes of Devotees

In Hindu Tantra, uniting the deity and the devotee uses meditation and ritual practices. These practices are divided among three classes of devotees: the animal, heroic, and the divine. In the divine devotee, the rituals are internal. The divine devotee is the only one who can attain the object of the rituals (awakening energy).

Doctrines

Defined as a technique-rich style of spiritual practice, Tantra has no single coherent doctrine; instead, it developed a variety of teachings in connection with the religions adopting the Tantric method. These practices are oriented to the married householder rather than the monastic or solitary renunciant, exhibiting a world-embracing (as opposed to a world-denying) character. Tantra, particularly its non-dual forms, rejected the values of Patañjalian yoga; instead, it offered a vision of reality as self-expression of a single, free and blissful divine consciousness under Œiva.

The World is Real

Since the world was seen as real (not illusory), this doctrine was an innovation on previous Indian philosophies (which saw the divine as transcendent and the world as illusion). The consequence of this view was that householders could aspire to spiritual liberation, where the lay practitioner addressed this goal by consulting Tantric manuals and undertaking various Tantric rituals.

Since Tantra dissolved the dichotomy between spiritual and mundane, practitioners could integrate their daily lives into their spiritual growth, seeking to realize the divine which is transcendent and immanent. Tantric practices and rituals aim to bring about a realization of the truth that "nothing exists that is not divine" (*nâúivamvidyate kvacit*), bringing freedom from ignorance and the cycle of suffering (*samsâra*).

Tantric visualizations are said to bring the meditator to the core of their humanity and unity with transcendence. Tantric meditations do not serve as training, extraneous beliefs or unnatural practices.

On the contrary, the transcendence reached by such meditative work does not construct anything in the mind of the practitioner; instead, it deconstructs all preconceived notions of the human condition. The limits on thought (cultural and linguistic frameworks) are removed. This allows the person to experience liberation, followed by unity with reality.

Evolution and Involution

According to Nikhilananda, "being-consciousness-bliss" (or *Satchidananda*) entails self-evolution and self-involution. *Prakriti* (reality) evolves into a multiplicity of things but also remains consciousness, being and bliss. *Maya* (illusion) veils reality, separating it into opposites (conscious and unconscious, pleasant and unpleasant). If not recognized as illusion, these opposing conditions limit (*pashu*) the individual *(jiva)*.

Shiva and Shakti are generally seen as distinct. Tantra affirms that the world and the individual *jiva* are real, distinguishing itself from dualism and the qualified non-dualism of Vedanta.

Evolution, or the "outgoing current," is only half of *Maya*. Involution (the "return current") takes the *jiva* back towards the source of reality, revealing the infinite. Tantra teaches the changing of the "outgoing current" into the "return current," removing the fetters of *Maya*. This view underscores two maxims of Tantra: "One must rise by that by which one falls," and "the very poison that kills becomes the elixir of life when used by the wise."

Texts

The primary sources of written Hindu Tantric lore are the *agama*, generally consisting of four parts: metaphysical knowledge (*jnana*), contemplative procedures (*yoga*), ritual regulations (*kriya*) and religious injunctions (*charya*). Tantric schools affiliate themselves with specific *agamic* traditions. Hindu tantra exists in *Shaiva, Vaisnava, Ganapatya, Saura* and *Shakta* forms, and individual tantric texts may be classified as *Shaiva Âgamas, Vaishnava Pâñcarâtra Samhitâs*, and *Shakta Tantras*. The word *Tantra* includes all such works. The religious culture of the Tantras is essentially Hindu, and Buddhist Tantric material can be shown to have been derived from Hindu sources.

Important texts in Tibetan Buddhism are the Kalachakra tantra and the Guhyasamâja tantra, both belonging to the

Anuttarayoga Tantra or Highest Yoga Tantra.

Tantras use twilight language (*sandhyâ-bhâshâ*), which makes them inaccessible for those who are not initiated. The term refers to the twilight, a "mysterious time of the day [which is] charged with power". It is a symbolic language, which both informs and illumines the practitioner by creating a rich symbolic context, and conceals the true meaning for those who are not initiated. It uses similes and paradoxes to describe the Tantric experiences and insights, for example *vajra* ("thunderbolt") = *linga* ("phallus") = *sunyata* ("empty" of an inherent essence).

Influence on Asian Religions

The Tantric method affected every major Indian religion during the early medieval period (c. 500–1200 CE); the Hindu sects of Shaivism, Shaktism, Vaishnavism and also Buddhism and Jainism developed a well-documented body of Tantric practices and doctrines, and Islam in India was also influenced by Tantra. Tantric ideas and practices spread from India to Tibet, Nepal, China, Japan, Cambodia, Vietnam and Indonesia. Tibetan Buddhism and some forms of Hinduism show the strongest Tantric influence, as do the postural yoga movement and most forms of American New Age spirituality.

Hinduism

Shaiva Tantra

The tantric Shaiva tradition consists of the Kapalikas, Kashmir Shaivism and Shaiva Siddhanta. The word "Tântrika" is used for followers of the Tantras in Shaivism.

Yoga

Shaiva tantra produced the Hatha Yoga manuals, such as the 15th-century Hathayoga Pradîpikâ and the 16th-century Gheranda Samhitâ, from which modern yoga derives. The earlier (pre-Tantric) form of yoga, dating back to the Yoga Sutras of Patanjali, became known as Raja Yoga: Yoga as it has been inherited in the modern world has its roots in

Tantric ritual and in secondary passages (pâdas) within Tantric scriptures. The practices of mantra, âsana (seat/pose), sense-withdrawal (pratyâhâra), breath-regulation (prânâyâma), mental (mantric) fixation (dhâranâ), meditation (dhyâna), mudrâ, the subtle body (sukshma shârîra) with its energy centers (chakras, âdhâras, granthis, etc.) and channels (nâdîs), as well as the phenomenon of Kundalinî Shakti are but a few of the tenets that comprise Tantric Yoga. While some of these derive from earlier, pre-Tantric sources, such as the Hindu Upanishads and the Yoga Sûtra, they were greatly expanded upon, ritualized, and philosophically contextualized in these medieval Tantras.

Vedic Tradition

Orthodox Brahmanas incorporate Tantric rituals into their daily activities (*ahnikas*). *Gayatri-avahanam* is a common element of Sandhyavandanam in southern India. Orthodox temple archakas of several sects follow rules laid out in Tantric texts; for example, priests of the Iyengar sect follow Pañcaratra *agamas*.

However, it has been claimed that orthodox Vedic traditions were inimical to Tantra. André Padoux notes that, in India, tantra rejects orthodox Vedic tenets. In his review of Tantric literature, Moriz Winternitz points out that while Indian Tantric texts are not hostile to the Vedas they see them as too difficult for the modern age. Many orthodox Brahmans who accept the authority of the Vedas reject the Tantras. Although later Tantric writers wanted to base their doctrines on the Vedas, some orthodox followers of the Vedic tradition denigrated Tantra as anti-Vedic.

Buddhist Tantra

The Tantric Buddhist tradition evolved in northern India and Nepal and later spread to Tibet and Mongolia where they are the dominant form of Buddhism. Vajrayana Buddhism includes scriptures written by the Indian Mahasiddhas. According to Tibetan Buddhist Tantric master Lama Thubten

Yeshe: ...each one of us is a union of all universal energy. Everything that we need in order to be complete is within us right at this very moment. It is simply a matter of being able to recognize it. This is the tantric approach.

In east Asia, there are various schools of Tantric Buddhism, or Tangmi. Tantric Buddhism arrived in China during the Tang dynasty and later reached Japan through the efforts of Kûkai (774–835) where it is known as Shingon Buddhism.

In Southeast Asia there is also a tradition called Tantric Theravada, particularly in Cambodia, where it was once the mainstream tradition. In the Indonesian islands of Java and Sumatra, Indonesian Esoteric Buddhism was also once dominant.

CHAPTER

2

Theism of Patanjali Sutra

Patañjali in YS I.23 states that the goal of Yoga can be attained by the grace of God, Ivara-pranidhanad va. The theistic, or Isvaravada element in Indic thought stretches back at least to the late Vedic period. Of the six "schools" of traditional thought that stem from this period, five - Nyâya, Vaisesika, Vedânta, Yoga and Sâmkhya - were, or became, theistic. Sâmkhya, although often represented as non-theistic, was, in point of fact, widely theistic in its early expressions, and continued to retain widespread theistic variants outside of the later classical philosophical school associated with Isvarakrsna, as evidenced in the Purânas and Bhagavad Gîtâ.

Reflecting Patañjali's undogmatic and non-sectarian sophistication, although Isvara-pranidhana, "devotion to God" may not be the exclusive or mandatory way to attain realisation of the self (given the particle va "or" in I.23) it is clearly favored by him. The term "Isvara" occurs in three distinct contexts in the Yoga Sûtras. The first, beginning with I.23, is in the context of how to attain the ultimate goal of Yoga, namely, the cessation of all thought, samprajñata samadhi and realisation of purusa. Patañjali presents dedication to Isvara as one such option. But it is important to note the word va, "or," in this sutra, indicating that Patañjali presents devotion to Isvara, the Lord, as an optional means of attaining samadhi, rather than an obligatory one.

In the ensuing discussion, Patañjali states that: the Lord is a special self because he is untouched by the deposits of samskaras, karma and its fructification, and the obstacles to the practice of yoga, the klesas of nescience, ego, attachment, aversion and the will-to-live. He is omniscient, and also the teacher of the ancients, because he is not limited by Time.

Given the primary context of the Sûtras, namely fixing the mind on an object, two sutras, I.27–28, specify how Isvara is to be meditated upon: "his designation is the mystical syllable "om," and its repetition, japa, and the contemplation of its meaning should be performed." This points to the ubiquitous and most prominent form of Hindu meditation from the classical period to the present day: mantra recitation (japa). As a result of this devotional type of meditation, "comes the realisation of the inner consciousness and freedom from all obstacles."

The second context in which Patañjali refers to Isvara is in the first sutra in chapter II, where kriya yoga, the path of action, is described as consisting of austerity, study and devotion to the Lord. By performing such kriya yoga, samadhi is attained and the obstacles, are weakened. The niyamas, which are the second limb of the eight-limbed path of Yoga, consist of cleanliness, contentment, austerity, study and, as in the other two contexts, Isvarapranidhana, devotion to Isvara (thus, the three ingredients of kriya yoga are all niyamas). The various benefits associated with following the yamas and niyamas, ethics and morals, are noted in the ensuing sutras of the chapter, and II.45 states that the benefit from the niyama of devotion to God is the attainment of samadhi. This is the final reference toIsvara in the text, but it is significant, because all the boons mentioned as accruing from the other yamas and niyamas(there are ten in all) represent prakrtic, or material, attainments - vitality, knowledge of past lives, detachment, etc., etc. It is only from Isvarapraridhana, the last item on the list of yamas andniyamas, that the ultimate goal of Yoga, samadhi, is achieved. These then are the gleanings that can be extracted from Patañjali's characteristically frugal sutras.

From these we can conclude that Patañjali is definitely promoting a degree of theistic practice in the Yoga Sûtras. Although in the first context, Isvarapranidhana, devotional surrender to God, is optional as a means of attaining samadhi, Patañjali does direct six sutras to Isvara, which is not insignificant given the frugality of his sutras.

This devotional surrender is not optional in the second context, kriya yoga. Since it is likewise not optional in the third context as a niyama, which is a prerequisite to meditational yoga, Patañjali seems to be requiring that all aspiring yogis be devotionally oriented in the preparatory stages to the higher goals of Yoga and, while in the higher, more meditational stages of practice they may shift their meditational focus of concentration to other objects - even, ultimately, to any object of their pleasing- they would best be advised to retain Isvara as object thereafter, since this "special purusa" can bestow perfection of samadhi which other objects cannot. Patañjali also states that Isvara is represented by the mystical syllable "om."

Om has been understood as a sonal incarnation of Brahman (which is the most common term used for the Absolute Truth in the Upanisads), since the late Vedic period.

A scholastic such as Patañjali would most certainly have been well schooled in the Upanisads, which, as an orthodox thinker, he would have accepted as sruti, divine revelation.

Even though he never refers to Brahman in the Sutras, here again we must wonder whether along with all the Isvara theologies of his time he is quite consciously equating the Upanisadic Brahman with this personal Isvara, by means of this common denominator of om.

It is through the sound om that the yogi is to fix the mind on Isvara. After all, since Isvara, as a type of purusa, is beyond prakrti, and therefore beyond conceptualisation or any type of vrtti, how is one to fix one's mind upon him - the prakrtic mind cannot perceive that which is finer than itself?

Patañjali here provides the means: through the recitation of the syllable in which Isvara manifests.

Such recitation is called japa (an old Vedic term common in the old Brâhmana texts, where it referred to the soft recitation of Vedic mantras by the priest.)

By constantly repeating omand contemplating its meaning, artha, namely Isvara, the mind of the yogi becomes one-pointed - the goal of all yoga practice. Repeating the sound om and "contemplating its meaning," namely, that it is the sound representation of Isvara, the object of the yogi's surrender, when coupled with Patañjali's usage of the word pranidhana, surrender, in I.23, points to chanting the mantra in a devotional mood. This is quintessential Hindu theistic meditation, the most prominent form of Hindu Yoga evidenced from antiquity to the present day.

YOGA: ITS ORIGIN, HISTORY AND DEVELOPMENT

The term 'Yoga' is derived from the Sanskrit root 'YUJ', meaning 'to join' or 'to yoke' or 'to unite'. As per Yogic scriptures the practice of Yoga leads to the union of individual consciousness with that of the Universal Consciousness, indicating a perfect harmony between the mind and body, Man and Nature. The aim of Yoga is Self-Realisation, to overcome all kinds of sufferings leading to 'the state of liberation'. This is one of the oldest sciences of the world, originated in India, which is very useful for preserving and maintaining one's physical and mental health and also for 'spiritual evolution'.

The practice of Yoga is believed to have started with the very dawn of civilization, Mythologically, the Lord Shiva is considered to be the first teacher of Yoga. Yoga, being widely considered as an 'immortal cultural outcome' of Indus valley civilization - dating back to 2700 B.C. - has proved itself catering to both material and spiritual upliftment of humanity.

Basic humane values are the very identity of Yoga Sadhana. The Number of seals and fossil remains of Indus valley civilization with Yogic motives and figures performing Yoga Sadhana suggest the presence of Yoga in ancient India. The phallic symbols, seals of idols of mother Goddess are suggestive of Tantra Yoga. Presence of Yoga is available in folk traditions, Indus valley civilization, Vedic and Upanishadic heritage, Buddhist and Jain traditions, Darshanas, epics of Mahabharat and Ramayana, theistic traditions of Shaivas, Vaishnavas, and Tantric traditions.

In addition, there was a primordial or pure Yoga which has been manifested in mystical traditions of South Asia. This was the time when Yoga was being practised under the direct guidance of Guru and its spritual value was given special importance. It was a part of Upasana and Yoga sadhana was inbuilt in their rituals. Sun was given highest importance during the vedic period. The practice of 'Surya namaskara' may have been invented later due to this influence. Pranayama was a part of daily ritual and to offer the oblation. Though Yoga was being practiced in the pre-Vedic period (2700 B.C.), the great Sage Maharshi Patanjali systematised and codified the then existing practices of Yoga, its meaning and its related knowledge through his Yoga Sutras. The philosophy and practice of Yoga itself was codified clearly and methodically by the sage Patanjali in his set of 196 aphorisms called "The Yoga Sutras". The Sutras bring together all the various strands of theory and practice of yoga and present them in one concise, integrated and comprehensive text. According to Patañjali, there are eight components of the practice referred to as Ashtanga Yoga or eight 'limbs' of Yoga sadhana which must be practised and refined in order to perceive the true self- the ultimate goal of Yoga.

Historical evidences of the existence of Yoga were seen in the pre-Vedic period (2700 B.C.), and thereafter till Patanjali's period. The main sources, from which we get the information about Yoga practices and the related literature during this period, are available in Vedas (4), Upanishads (108), Smritis, teachings of Buddhism, Jainism, Panini, Epics (2), Puranas (18) etc. Tentatively, the period between 500 BC - 800 A.D. is considered as the Classical period which is also considered as the most fertile and prominent period in the history and development of Yoga. During this period, commentaries of Vyasa on Yoga Sutras and Bhagawadgita etc. came into existence.This period can be mainly dedicated to two great religious teachers of India – Mahavir and Buddha. The concept of Five great vows - Pancha mahavrata - by Mahavir and Ashta Magga or eight-fold path by Buddha - can be well considered as early nature of Yoga sadhana. We find its more explicit explanation in Bhagawadgita which has elaborately presented the concept of Gyan Yoga, Bhakti Yoga and Karma Yoga. These three types of Yoga are still the highest example of human wisdom and and even to day people find peace by following the methods as shown in Gita. Patanjali's Yoga sutra besides containing various aspects of Yoga, is mainly identified with eight fold path of Yoga.

The very important commentary on Yoga sutra by Vyasa was also written. During this very period the aspect of mind was given importance and it was clearly brought out through Yoga sadhana, Mind and body both can be brought under control to experience equanimity. The period between 800 A.D. - 1700 A.D. has been recognised as the Post-classical period wherein the teachings of great Acharyatrayas - Adi Shankracharya, Ramanujacharya, Madhavacharya - were prominent during this period. The teachings of Surdas, Tulasidas, Purandardas, Mirabai were the great contributors during this period. The Natha Yogis of Hathayoga Tradition like Matsyendranatha, Gorkshanatha, Cauranginatha, Swatmaram Suri, Gheranda, Shrinivasa Bhatt are some of the great personalities who popularised the Hatha Yoga practices during this period.

The period between 1700 - 1900 A.D. is considered as Modern period in which the great Yogacharyas - Ramana

Maharshi, Ramakrishna Paramhansa, Paramhansa Yogananda, Vivekananda etc. have contributed for the development of Raja Yoga. This was the period when Vedanta, Bhakti yoga, Nathayoga or Hatha-Yoga flourished. The Shadanga-yoga of Goraksha shatakam, Chaturanga-yoga of Hathayoga pradipika, Saptanga-yoga of Gheranda Samhita were the main tenents of Hatha-yoga. Now in the contemporary times, everybody has conviction about yoga practices towards the preservation, maintenance and promotion of health. Yoga has spread all over the world by the teachings of great personalities like Swami Shivananda, Shri T. Krishnamacharya, Swami Kuvalayananda, Shri Yogendara, Swami Rama, Sri Aurobindo, Maharshi Mahesh Yogi, Acharya Rajanish, Pattabhijois, BKS. Iyengar, Swami Satyananda Sarasvati and the like. These different Philosophies, Traditions, lineages and Guru-shishya paramparas of Yoga lead to the emergence of differnt Traditional Schools of Yoga *e.g.* Jnana-yoga, Bhakti-yoga, Karma-yoga, Dhyana-yoga, Patanjala-yoga, Kundalini-yoga, Hatha-yoga, Mantra-yoga, Laya-yoga, Raja-yoga, Jain-yoga, Bouddha-yoga etc. Each school has its own principles and practices leading to altimate aim and objectives of Yoga.

However, the widely practiced Yoga Sadhanas (Practices) are: Yama, Niyama, Asana, Pranayama, Pratyahara, Dharana, Dhyana (Meditation), Samadhi/ Samyama, Bandhas and Mudras, Shat-karmas, Yukta-ahara, Yukta karma, Mantra japa etc. Yama's are restraints and Niyama's are observances. These are considered to be pre-requisits for the Yoga Sadhanas (Practices).

Asanas, capable of bringing about stability of body and mind 'kuryat-tad-asanam-sthairyam...', consists in adopting various body (psycho-physical) patterns, giving ability to maintain a body position (a stable awareness of one's structural existence) for a considerable length and period of time as well. Pranayama consists in developing awareness of one's breathing followed by willful regulation of respiration as the functional or vital basis of one's existence. It helps in developing awareness of one's mind and helps to establish control over the mind.

In the initial stages, this is done by developing awareness of the 'flow of in-breath and out-breath' (svasa-prasvasa) through nostrils, mouth and other body openings, its internal and external pathways and destinations. Later, this phenomenan is modified, through regulated, controlled and monitored inhalation (svasa) leading to the awareness of the body space/s getting filled (puraka), the space/s remaning in a filled state (kumbhaka) and it's getting emptied (rechaka) during regulated, controlled and monitored exhalation (prasvasa). Pratyahara indicates dissociation of one's consciousness (withdrawal) from the sense organs which helps one to remain connected with the external objects. Dharana indicates broad based field of attetion (inside the body and mind) which is usually understood as concentration. Dhyana (Meditation) is contemplation (focussed attention inside the body and mind) and Samadhi - integration.

Bandhas and Mudras are practices associated with pranayama. They are viewed as (the) higher Yogic practices mainly consisting on adopting certain body (psycho-physical) patterns along with (as well as) control over respiration.This further facilitates control over mind and paves way for higher yogic attainment. Shat-karmas are de-toxification procedures, help to remove the toxins acumalated in the body and are clinical in nature.Yuktahara (Right Food and other inputs) advocates appropriate food and food habits for healthy living. However practice of Dhyana (Meditation) helping in self-realisation leading to transcendence is considered as the esssence of Yoga Sadhana (The Practice of Yoga).

Traditionally, Yoga Education was imparted by knowledgeable, experienced, and wise persons in the families (comparable with the education imparted in convents in the west) and then by the Seers (Rishis/ Munis/ Acharyas) in Ashramas (compared with monastries). Yoga Education, on the other hand, aims at taking care of the individual, the

'Being'. It is presumed that a good, balanced, integrated, truthful, clean, transparent person will be more useful to oneself, family, society, nation, nature and humanity at large. Yoga education is 'Being oriented'. Details of working with 'being oriented' aspect have been outlined in various living traditions and texts and the method contributing to this important field is known as 'Yoga'.

Present days, Yoga Education is being imparted by many eminent Yoga Institutions, Yoga Colleges, Yoga Universites, Yoga Departments in the Universities, Naturopathy colleges and Private trusts and societies. Many Yoga Clinics, Yoga Therapy and Training Centers, Preventive Health Care Units of Yoga, Yoga Research Centers etc. have been established in Hospitals, Dispensories, Medical Institiutions and Therapetical setups.

Different social customs and rituals in India, the land of Yoga, reflect a love for ecological balance, tolerance towards other systems of thought and a compassionate outlook towards all creations.Yoga Sadhana of all hues and colours is considered panacea for a meaningful life and living. Its orientation to a comprehensive health, both individual and social, makes it a worthy practice for the people of all religions, races and nationalities. With the wide spread popularity of Yoga around the globe has culminated in the development of several modern schools or styles of Yoga, which includes Astanga, Ananda, Bihar, Bikram, Integral, Iyengar, Kripalu, Kundalini, Sivananda, Vini-yoga, Vinyas, Art of Living, Vipassana, Preksha and Transcendental Meditation.

Particular styles or methods may be considered more effective than others or may suit an individual's temperament better. That said, it must always be remembered that all these are merely different methods of reaching for the same ultimate goal. They are all aspects of the overall philosophy of Yoga and, by and large, variations of 'Hatha Yoga' which rests on a strong foundation of physical techniques to enable the journey towards the union of body, breath and mind. Although Yoga Practice is essential for self realisation, it is also widely used for management of several diseases.

Conventional medical management of many conditions is proving to be inadequate and inefficient and, increasingly, medical professionals are happy to try alternative and complementary therapies including Yoga. Who has recognised Yoga as one of several traditional therapeutic systems originates in India and Yoga training and therapy departments are being opened in reputed, established medical Institutions and hospitals. Daily life in the modern world has left us with an immobile, sedentary lifestyle. This lack of exercise in our lives has left many people with chronic health and stress problems, especially as they get older. Yoga enables the practitioner to find relief from these physical ailments and to strengthen the body and make it suppler. It is particularly beneficial for - muscular-skeletal disorders, arthritis, pains in the knees, shoulders and other joints, curvatures of the back and back pain, slipped discs and sciatic pain. From the psychological viewpoint, Yoga practice smoothen emotions, sharpens the intellect and aids concentration and steadies the emotions.

Yoga can be used to manage stress, psycho-somatic and lifestyle related disorders. Non-communicable diseases very well respond to the Yoga therapy. The modern medicine Hospitals and Institutes are gradually adopting this system of therapy as an adjuvant care along with the conventional medical care and such Hospitals have started exclusive Centers for Yoga in their Hospitals/ Institutes. This trend is growing. Yoga departments in various colleges and universities and the integration of Yoga education in school curriculum and other institutionalised courses have played a vital role in the advancement and spread of Yoga. Yoga Demonstrations, Yoga conferences, seminars, workshops, exhibitions, magazines and journals have also contributed immensely to the popularity of this discipline.

With the advent of technology, Yoga is being promulgated via T.V. channels and the internet. Apart from this, publication of manuscripts, translations of critical editions of old authoritative texts and literature in different languages, articles based on laboratory studies and findings have ensured that the philosophy and practice of Yoga cross the shores of India. Yoga is becoming more and more relevant in today's conflict ridden world, providing strength and equanimity to mankind to face the challenges of the present and future and create a compassionate world. This is its greatest contribution to mankind in general and to the Cultural Heritage of India, in particular. Traditionally, the 'Guru' was accepting all the responsibility to initiate, educate, guide and take care of the welfare of the aspsirants, disciples and the students (sadhakas). There were different Gurus to initiate and guide different groups of people. In this respect, different yoga protocols developed for different mentalities and behaviour patterns will be viable in the changed circumstances with different paradigms.

MEANING AND PURPOSE OF THE YOGA SUTRAS

Yoga means Union and the purpose is to teach the practitioner of Yoga, called the Yogi, how to achieve Union or Spiritual Absorption into the Supreme Absolute or God. Yoga teachs us that our true self is the soul and that our self identity is an illusion to be overcome. These sutras do not go into the specifics of meditation, such as how to sit, what postures are best, etc... because it was assumed this material would be taught by a teacher to a student and that certain basics would be part of the instruction. It is recommended that the reader become famailiar with basic meditation techniques and postures before practicing these precepts.

Organisation of the Yoga Sutras

These sutras are in four parts (padas):

- *Samadhi Pada I:* Contemplation and Meditation

- *Sadhana Pada II:* The Steps To Union
- *Vibhuti Pada III:* Union Achieved And Its Results
- *Kaivalya Pada IV:* Illumination and Freedom.

Notes on this Translation of the Yoga Sutras

The Yoga Sutras of Patanjali were originally written in Sanskrit which is an Indo-European language. Sankrit is the oldest of the Indo-European languages still in active use. It is closely related to ancient Greek, Latin, Avestan and many other languages. It is the mother of Hindi/Urdu, Bengali, Gujarati, Punjabi, Marathi, Nepali, Simhal(Srilanka) and many other languages. Many Indian and Asian languages use a large number of Sanskrit words. Ancient texts of Hindus of various traditions, Buddhists, Jains and Sikhs are in Sanskrit or related languages (Pali/Prakrit/Hindi). The language of Zoroastrian Avesta is a dialect of the Vedic Sanskrit. The word Sanskrit itself mean 'perfected polished literature' and is a highly organised language with a complex grammer.

It is very difficult to translate Sanskrit to English with a word for word literal equality. Many translations attempt to bypass this difficulty in two ways. One is to not translate certain words but to leave them in their anglicised spelling, whereas the reader is expected to learn the definition of the word. Another way the translator will transcend the problem will be to add commentaries further explaining each sentence or phrase. Both systems can be cumbersome to the reader.

This translation does not attempt word for word equality, instead translates each sanskrit word compound to an equivalent English phrase or word pair. This prevents burdening the reader with unfamiliar words or cumbersome commentary.

Also certain words should be recognised as to their intent and meaning. In typical English translations of Yoga concepts, the word Consciousness is frequently used. This word is imprecise when used in the context that Patanjali taught. In this translation the word Awareness is used as it more precisely delivers the meaning Patanjali intended sinceConsciousness has a connotation of mind and awareness in modern English, whereas Awareness is a more basic, purer concept.

Other important terms used here is the word integration or words meditative integration. In the context of the Yoga Sutras, this word refers to concentration, meditation, and spiritual absorption, jointly together, and is a key concept most translations render as samyama.

The words seer, meditator and Yogi can be considered equivalent in this text. Attempts have been made to render the text gender neutral, where it was too awkward the pronoun he or his is used.

ETHICS OF PATANJALI SUTRA

Verse I.33 states that as a result of cultivating an attitude of "friendship" with those who find themselves in a "situation of happiness," one of "compassion" towards those in "distress," one of "joy" towards "pious" selves, and one of "equanimity" or indifference towards the "impious," sattva is generated. Consequently, the mind becomes lucid - clarity being the nature of sattva. Once clear, one-pointed concentration, or steadiness, which is the goal of meditational Yoga, can be achieved by the mind.

From an ethical point of view, by being a well-wisher towards those who are happy, as well as those who are virtuous, the contamination of envy is removed. By compassion towards those miserable, that is, by wishing to remove someone's miseries as if they were one's own, the contamination of the desire to inflict harm on others is removed.

By equanimity towards the impious, the contamination of intolerance is removed. By thus removing these traits of envy, desire to inflict harm, and intolerance, which are characteristics of rajas and tamas, the sattva natural to the mind can manifest. In the ensuing state of lucidity, the inclination towards seeking higher truths by controlling the vrttis, in other words towards cultivating a focused state of mind by the practice ofyoga, spontaneously arises, because the inclination for enlightenment is natural to the pure sattvic mind.

A further set of ethical practices indispensable for increasing the sattva component of the mind are the five yamas, observances (literally "restraints") of chapter II: non-violence, truthfulness; refrainment from stealing; celibacy and renunciation of [unnecessary] possessions. From these,ahimsa, non-violence, is the yama singled out by the commentators for special attention, and therefore leads the list and thus, the entire eight limbs of Yoga (it seems important to note that theyamas themselves lead the list of the eight limbs suggesting that one's yogic accomplishment remains limited until the yamas are internalised and put into practice). Vyâsa accordingly takes ahimsa as the root of the other yamas. He defines it as not injuring any living creature anywhere at any time. Just as the footprints of an elephant covers the footprints of all other creatures, so does ahimsa cover all the other yamas - one continues to undertake more and more vows and austerities for the sole purpose of purifying ahimsa.

Vyâsa defines "truth," the second yama, as one's words and thoughts being in exact correspondence to fact, that is, to whatever is known through the three processes of knowledge accepted by the Yoga school. Speech is for the transfer of one's knowledge to others, and should not be deceitful, misleading or devoid of value. It should be for the benefit of all creatures, and not for their harm. However, underscoring the centrality of ahimsa – truth must never result in violence. In other words, if there is ever a conflict between the yamas – if observing one yama results in the compromise of another – then ahimsa must always be respected first.

"Refrainment from stealing," the third yama, is described as not taking things belonging to others, and not even harboring the desire to do so. Vyâsa defines "celibacy" as the control of the sexual organs, and this is further refined by Vâcaspati Miúra as not seeing, speaking with, embracing, or otherwise interacting with members of the opposite sex as objects of desire. In short, self-realisation cannot be attained if one is sexually absorbed because this indicates that one is still seeking fulfillment on the sensual level, and thus misidentifying with the non-self.

Vyâsa defines "renunciation of possessions" as the ability to see the problems caused by the acquisition, preservation and destruction of things, since these only provoke attachment and injury. These yamas are considered the great vow; they are not exempted by one's class, place, time or circumstance. They are universal in all aspects of life's affairs and social interactions. Without them rajas and tamas cannot be curtailed, and the sattva essential to the higher stages of Yoga is unattainable.

CHAPTER

3

Philosophical Foundation of Patanjali's Yoga Sutra

The science of yoga is very ancient. However, the first systematic exposition of yoga was made by Patanjali in his famous Yogasutra. He expounds, in very clear and systematic manners, the techniques of yoga, which, for him, are primarily psychological though mixed with some physical practices like asana and pranayam in the beginning. In the primary sense, yoga means samadhi as it is signified by the definition yogas-citta-vrtti-nirodhah and so, the other practices are only the limbs of it. This state of yoga is not adventitious but natural to the mind sarva-bhaumas-cittasya dharmah since it is evolved from the sattva aspect as it is rightly pointed out by his commentator. The culmination of yoga is the state of asamprajnata or nirbija samadhi where the seer, drasta, remains in his own natural state of being or svarupa, whereas in other states, it gets identified with the modifications of the mind.

Patanjali bases his yoga on the philosophical framework of Sankhya. Since his primary aim is to expound yoga he does not explain the philosophical concepts which are taken for granted as established facts. It is conspicuous that yoga is an ancient spiritual practice. Though it is mainly sadhana-intensive, it has a well defined conceptual basis without which it cannot happen. We find different types of yoga as hatha yoga, kundalini yoga, raja yoga etc, which are based on different concepts.

The Advaita Vedanta School adopts yoga in its non-dualistic framework where it has a secondary place since the primary aim is to dispel ignorance which blurs the knowledge of the Self through vicara.The Agama schools have their own concepts of mantra, kundalini, six cakras like muladhara etc, with practices which are peculiar to their world view. The Hatha yoga School which adopts the same concepts as kundalini, sat cakra etc, is more prominent for its giving emphasis on the physical body where as its world view is akin to that of the Agamic schools. In Advaita Vedanta, the world is said to be a false appearance or vivarta and the Self is the same as Brahman, the Reality which is the substratum of the cosmic appearance. So there is neither attainment of a new state nor a negation of an old one. In the Agamic view, there is a real attainment, the merger of the individual with the Universal Self, God. Even though the main stream Agamic view is non-dualistic, the world is not taken as false, since, unlike Advaita Vedanta, the Agamic schools do not accept vivarta vada. For Patanjali, like Sankhya, yoga is the state of the Self where it remains completely isolated from Prakrti. It is described as the establishment of citsakti in its own svarupa.

Different schools adopt yoga and mould it to their philosophic framework. Even though concepts and practices are different the underlying spirit and mechanism remain the same. The main standpoint is to discipline the body and the mind so that one can explore deeper levels of his own being which remain hidden in ordinary states of existence. It is the common experience that our knowledge extends over to the objects in the ordinary states inclusive of both valid and invalid knowledge. Otherwise, the mind lapses into sleep. These are the states which Patanjali classifies into five vrttis, valid knowledge, erroneous knowledge, sleep and the rest. Never, in the ordinary level, do we encounter any state of mind beyond these five vrttis. But the state beyond them is the starting point where yoga begins. The possibility of a state of consciousness beyond the five states of mind is plausible in view of the fact that the Self is accepted as different from mind by the Indian systems of philosophy. The Upanisads describe a fourth state of consciousness beyond waking, dream and deep sleep. The impurities which are accumulated around the mind and the senses can be got rid of only when one discovers him to be different from them. This conception of the Self which gives a sense of transcendence provides the metaphysical background of the science of yoga in whichever framework it might have developed. It is obvious that Sankhya-Yoga, Vedanta and the Agamic Schools which develop their philosophical ideas around such a conception provide the most favourable background for the most remarkable spiritual traditions in India.

The foundational ideas of Patanjali's yoga can be summed up in a few lines. The seer, the subject is essentially pure consciousness who only sees through the modifications of the mind. Patanjali remains silent on the question whether this pure consciousness is also the same or a part of the universal consciousness if at all such a reality is accepted. Even though Isvara, God is accepted as omniscient, untouched by miseries, actions and their results etc, his causal relation with the individual is not explained.

Patanjali accepts a sort of realism where the objective world, drsya is real. He upholds citta, mind-stuff as a separate principle which being tinged by both the object and the Self gives rise to empirical knowledge. The mind is coloured by innumerable impressions with which the purusa identifies him and is entangled in the enjoyments of the world. Through discrimination the purusa becomes free from such entanglements. Then the gunas being bereft any purpose for the purusa get dissolved inversely in their primordial cause which is known as kaivalya, the state of freedom of the purusa, where he gets established in his own svarupa. The mind which is the cause of the samsara is also the means of freedom when it is oriented towards the Self through discrimination. The process of the world is intended to facilitate the evolution of the purusa towards his self-attainment, which is isolation from prakrti otherwise known as kaivalya.

The theory of plurality of purusas is not compatible with the conception of purusa as nitya and bibhu. The state of kaivalya in the scheme of Sankhya cannot consistently explain many metaphysical questions. It cannot explain the state of the purusa with reference to the real space, time and the cosmos after the attainment of kaivalya. It is not worthwhile to yearn for kaivalya which is simply a state of inactivity as that of the pralayakala or the vijnanakala of the Agamas or that of the mukta of the Vaisesikas. Patanjali has adopted Sankhya as a philosophical model for his more practical science of yoga, but he has something more to say which becomes conspicuous from his description of the final samadhi as dharmamegha and his contention that knowledge, free from all concealment surpasses infinitely all knowable at the final stage of enlightenment.

The state of enlightenment or freedom as the consummation of the process of life is not easy to conceive. It is even more difficult to explain. Patanjali's yoga leads the sadhaka along the path of enlightenment till its accomplishment. But as a final world view the non-dualistic standpoint of Vedanta is philosophically more satisfying. Patanjali's yoga can very well be incorporated within the Vedantic philosophy of non-dualism.

Indeed, Vidyaranya Swami, the illustrious writer of Pancadasi opines in this line - "From the worshippers of God in form of a small grass to the followers of Yoga, all have a wrong idea about Isvara. From the Lokayatas, the materialists to the followers of Sankhya, all have confusion regarding the jiva."Then he adds -"If the conceptions of plurality of jivas, the reality of the world and the difference of God and jiva are given up, then there will be a grand synthesis of Sankhya, Yoga and Vedanta"

YOGA SUTRAS OF PATANJALI

In Indian philosophy, Yoga is the name of one of the six orthodox philosophical schools. The Yoga philosophical system is closely allied with the Samkhya school. The Yoga school as expounded by Patanjali accepts the Samkhya psychology and metaphysics, but is more theistic than the Samkhya, as evidenced by the addition of a divine entity to the Samkhya's twenty-five elements of reality.

The parallels between Yoga and Samkhya were so close that Max Muller says that "the two philosophies were in popular parlance distinguished from each other as Samkhya with and Samkhya without a Lord...." The intimate relationship between Samkhya and Yoga is explained by Heinrich Zimmer:

These two are regarded in India as twins, the two aspects of a single discipline. Sankhya provides a basic theoretical exposition of human nature, enumerating and defining its elements, analyzing their manner of cooperation in a state of bondage (bandha), and describing their state of disentanglement or separation in release (moksa), while Yoga treats specifically of the dynamics of the process for the disentanglement, and outlines practical techniques for the gaining of release, or 'isolation-integration' (kaivalya).

The sage Patanjali is regarded as the founder of the formal Yoga philosophy. The Yoga Sutras of Patanjali are ascribed to Patanjali, who, may have been, as Max Muller explains, "the author or representative of the Yoga-philosophy without being necessarily the author of the Sutras." Indologist Axel Michaels is dismissive of claims that the work was written by Patanjali, characterizing it instead as a collection of fragments and traditions of texts stemming from the second or third century. Gavin Flood cites a wider period of uncertainty for the composition, between 100 BC and 500 CE.

Patanjali's yoga is known as Raja yoga, which is a system for control of the mind. Patanjali defines the word "yoga" in his second sutra, which is the definitional sutra for his entire work:

yogas citta-vitti-nirodha?-Yoga Sutras 1.2

This terse definition hinges on the meaning of three Sanskrit terms. I. K. Taimni translates it as "Yoga is the inhibition (nirodha?) of the modifications (v?tti) of the mind (citta)".

Swami Vivekananda translates the sutra as "Yoga is restraining the mind-stuff (Citta) from taking various forms (Vrittis)." Gavin Flood translates the sutra as "yoga is the cessation of mental fluctuations".

Patanjali's writing also became the basis for a system referred to it as "Ashtanga Yoga" ("Eight-Limbed Yoga"). This eight-limbed concept derived from the 29th Sutra of the 2nd book became a feature of Raja yoga, and is a core characteristic of practically every Raja yoga variation taught today. The Eight Limbs of yoga practice are:

(1) Yama (The five "abstentions"): violence, lying, theft, (illicit) sex, and possessions
(2) Niyama (The five "observances"): purity, contentment, austerities, study, and surrender to god
(3) Asana: Literally means "seat", and in Patanjali's Sutras refers to seated positions used for meditation. Later, with the rise of Hatha yoga, asana came to refer to all the "postures"
(4) Pranayama ("Life Force Control"): Control of prana, life force, or vital energy, particularly, the breath
(5) Pratyahara ("Abstraction"): Reversal of the sense organs
(6) Dharana ("Concentration"): Fixing the attention on a single object
(7) Dhyana ("Meditation"): Intense contemplation of the nature of the object of meditation
(8) Samadhi ("Liberation"): merging consciousness with the object of meditation

It details every aspect of the meditative process, and the preparation for it. The book is available in as many as 40 English translations, both in-print and on-line.

HATHA YOGA PRADIPIKA

Hatha Yoga is a particular system of Yoga described by Yogi Swatmarama, a yogic sage of the 15th century in India, and compiler of the Hatha Yoga Pradipika. Hatha Yoga is a development of-but also differs substantially from-the Raja Yoga of Patanjali, in that it focuses on shatkarma, the purification of the physical as leading to the purification of the mind (ha) and prana, or vital energy (tha).

In contrast, the Raja Yoga posited by Patanjali begins with a purification of the mind (yamas) and spirit (niyamas), then comes to the body via asana (body postures) and pranayama (breath). Hatha yoga contains substantial tantric influence, and marks the first point at which chakras and kundalini were introduced into the yogic canon. Compared to the seated Asanas of Patanjali's Raja yoga which were seen largely as a means of preparing for meditation, it also marks the development of Asanas as full body 'postures' in the modern sense. Hatha Yoga in its many modern variations is the style that most people actually associate with the word "Yoga" today. Because its emphasis is on the body through asana and pranayama practice, many western students are satisfied with the physical health and vitality it develops and are not interested in the other six limbs of the complete Hatha yoga teaching, or with the even older Raja Yoga tradition it is based on.

Yoga in other Traditions

Yoga and Buddhism: Yoga is intimately connected to the religious beliefs and practices of the Indian religions. The influence of Yoga is also visible in Buddhism, which is distinguished by its austerities, spiritual exercises, and trance states.

Yogacara Buddhism

Yogacara also spelled yogachara, is a school of philosophy and psychology that developed in India during the 4th to 5th centuries. Yogacara received the name as it provided a yoga, a framework for engaging in the practices that lead to the path of the bodhisattva. The Yogacara sect teaches yoga in order to reach enlightenment.

Zen (Ch`an) Buddhism

Zen (the name of which derives from the Sanskrit "dhyana" via the Chinese "ch'an") is a form of Mahayana Buddhism. The Mahayana school of Buddhism is noted for its proximity with Yoga. In the west, Zen is often set alongside Yoga; the two schools of meditation display obvious family resemblances. This phenomenon merits special attention since the Zen Buddhist school of meditation has some of its roots in yogic practices. Certain essential elements of Yoga are important both for Buddhism in general and for Zen in particular.

Tibetan Buddhism

Yoga is central to Tibetan Buddhism. In the Nyingma tradition, practitioners progress to increasingly profound levels of yoga, starting with Maha yoga, continuing to Anu yoga and ultimately undertaking the highest practice, Ati yoga. In the Sarma traditions, the Anuttara yoga class is equivalent. Other tantra yoga practices include a system of 108 bodily postures practised with breath and heart rhythm. Timing in movement exercises is known as Trul khor or union of moon and sun (channel) prajna energies. The body postures of Tibetan ancient yogis are depicted on the walls of the Dalai Lama's summer temple of Lukhang.

Yoga and Tantra

Tantrism, is a practice that is supposed to alter the relation of the individual practitioner of Tantrism to the ordinary social, religious, and logical reality in which he or she lives. Through Tantric practice an individual perceives reality as maya, illusion, and the individual achieves liberation from it. This particular path to salvation among the several offered by Hinduism, links Tantrism to those practices of Indian religions, such as yoga, meditation, and social renunciation, which are based on temporary or permanent withdrawal from social relationships and modes.

During tantric practices and studies, the student is instructed further in meditation technique, particularly chakra meditation. This is often in a limited form in comparison with the way this kind of meditation is known and used by Tantric practitioners and yogis elsewhere, but is more elaborate than the initiate's previous meditation. It is considered to be a kind of Kundalini Yoga for the purpose of moving the Goddess into the chakra located in the "heart," for meditation and worship.

Goal of Yoga

There are numerous opinions on what the goal of Yoga may be, although generally they involve some kind of union, either of a personal or a non-personal nature.

Within the monist schools of Advaita Vedanta and Shaivism this perfection takes the form of Moksha, which is a liberation from all worldly suffering and the cycle of birth and death (Samsara) at which point there is a cessation of thought and an experience of blissful union with the Supreme Brahman. For the dualistic bhakti schools of Vaishnavism, bhakti itself is the ultimate goal of the yoga process, wherein perfection culminates in an eternal relationship with Vishnu or one of his associated avatars such as Krishna or Rama.

DHARANA

Dharana is a Sanskrit term from the verbal root dhri to hold, carry, maintain, resolve; and it is the sixth stage, step or limb of eight elucidated by Patanjali's Ashtanga Yoga or Raja Yoga. For a detailed account of the Eight Limbs, refer to the Yoga Sutras of Patanjali.

Dharana may be translated as "holding", "holding steady", "concentration" or "single focus". The prior limb Pratyahara invoves withdrawing the senses from external phenomena. Dharana builds further upon this by refining it further to ekagrata or ekagra chitta, that is single-pointed concentration and focus, which is in this context cognate with shamata. Maehle (2006: p.234) defines Dharana as: "The mind thinks about one object and avoids other thoughts; awareness of the object is still interrupted."

Dharana is the initial step of deep concentrative meditation, where the object being focused upon is held in the mind without consciousness wavering from it. The difference between Dharana, Dhyana, and Samadhi is that in the former, the object of meditation, the meditator, and the act of meditation itself remain separate.

That is, the meditator or the meditator's meta-awareness is conscious of meditating (that is, is conscious of the act of meditation) on an object, and of his or her own self, which is concentrating on the object. In the subsequent stage of Dhyana, as the meditator becomes more advanced, consciousness of the act of meditation disappears, and only the consciousness of being/existing and the object of concentration exist (in the mind).

DHYANA

Dhyana in Sanskrit or Jhana in Pali refers to a type or aspect of meditation. It is a key concept in Hinduism and Buddhism. Equivalent terms are "Chan" in modern Chinese, "Zen" in Japanese, "Seon" in Korea, and Samten in Tibetan.

Dhyana in Hinduism

In Hinduism, dhyana is considered to be an instrument to gain self knowledge, separating maya from reality to help attain the ultimate goal of Moksha.

The Bhagavad Gita, thought to have been written some time between 400 and 100 BC, talks of four branches of yoga:

- *Karma yoga:* The yoga of action in the world
- *Jnana yoga:* The yoga of Wisdom and intellectual endeavour
- *Bhakti yoga:* The yoga of devotion to God
- *Dhyana yoga*: The yoga of meditation

Dhyana in Raja Yoga is also found in Patanjali's Yoga Sutras. Depictions of Hindu yogis performing dhyana are found in ancient texts and in statues and frescoes of ancient India temples.

Dhyana in Buddhism

In the Theravada Tradition: In the Pali Canon the Buddha describes four progressive states of absorption meditation or jhana. The jhanas are said by the Buddha to be conducive to detachment but they must not be mistaken for the final goal of nibbana. The jhanas are states of meditation where the mind is free from the five hindrances (craving, aversion, sloth, agitation, doubt) and incapable of discursive thinking. The deeper jhanas can last for many hours. When a meditator emerges from jhana, his/her mind is empowered and able to penetrate into the deepest truths of existence.

There are four deeper states of meditative absorption called the immaterial attainments. Sometimes these are also referred to as the "formless" jhanas, or arupajhana (distinguished from the first four jhanas, rupajhana). In the Buddhist canonical texts, the word jhana is never explicitly used to denote them, but they are always mentioned in sequence after the first four jhanas.

Jhanas are normally described according to the nature of the mental factors which are present in these states

1. Movement of the mind onto the object, Vitakka (Sanskrit: Vitarka)
2. Retention of the mind on the object, Vicara
3. Joy, Piti (Sanskrit: Priti)
4. Happiness, Sukha

5. Equanimity, Upekkha (Sanskrit: Upekna)
6. One-pointedness, Ekaggata (Sanskrit: Ekagrata)

First Jhana (Vitakka, Vicara, Piti, Sukha, Ekaggata)

The five hindrances have completely disappeared and intense unified bliss remains. Only the subtlest of mental movement remains-perceivable in its absence by those who have entered the second jhana. The ability to form unwholesome intentions ceases.

Second Jhana (Piti, Sukha, Ekaggata)

All mental movement utterly ceases. There is only bliss. The ability to form wholesome intentions cease as well.

Third Jhana (Sukha, Ekaggata)

One half of bliss disappears (joy).

Fourth Jhana (Upekkha, Ekaggata)

The other half of bliss (happiness) disappears, leading to a state with neither pleasure nor pain, which the Buddha said is actually a subtle form of happiness (more sublime than piti and sukha). The Buddha described the jhanas as "the footsteps of the tathagata". The breath is said to cease temporarily in this state.

Traditionally, this fourth jhana is seen as the beginning of attaining psychic powers (abhigna).

The scriptures state that one should not seek to attain ever higher jhanas but master one first, then move on to the next. 'Mastery of jhana' involves being able to enter a jhana at will, stay as long as one likes, leave at will and experience each of the jhana factors as required. They also seem to suggest that lower jhana factors may manifest themselves in higher jhanas, if the jhanas have not been properly developed. The Buddha is seen to advise his disciples to concentrate and steady the jhana further.

In Mahayana traditions

In the Mahayana tradition, dhyana is the fifth of six

paramitas (perfections). It is usually translated as "concentration" or "meditative stability."

In East Asia, several schools of Buddhism were founded that focused on dhyana, under the names Chan, Zen, and Seon. According to tradition, Bodhidharma brought Dhyana to the Shaolin Temple in China, where it came to be transliterated as "chan" ("seon" in Korea, and then "zen" in Japan).

Dhyana in Jainism is called Samayika.

SAMADHI

Samadhi is a Hindu and Buddhist term that describes a non-dualistic state of consciousness in which the consciousness of the experiencing subject becomes one with the experienced object, and in which the mind becomes still (one-pointed or concentrated) though the person remains conscious. Sahaj samadhi is the effortless and continual state of perfection of a satguru. It varies from technical terms used to describe the higher levels of concentrated meditation, or dhyana (alt. "jhana"), in Yogic schools, and is considered a precursor for enlightenment, or Nirvana, in Buddhism. It is the eighth and final limb of the Yoga Sutra of Patanjali, and comprises the pinnacle of achievements in Samyama, the three-tiered practice of meditation including also dharana and dhyana.

Samadhi is also the Hindi word for a structure commemorating the dead (similar to a mausoleum), which may or may not contain the body of the deceased. Samadhis are often built in this way to honour people regarded as saints or gurus in Hindu religious traditions wherein such souls are said to have passed into (or were already in) samadhi at the time of death.

Etymology

Samadhi is a Sanskrit term for the state of consciousness induced by complete meditation. Its etymology comes from sam (together or integrated), a (towards), and dha (to get, to hold). Thus the result might be seen to be to acquire integration or wholeness, or truth (samapatti).

Samadhi in Hinduism

Samadhi is the main subject of the first part of the Yoga Sutras called Samadhi-pada. According to Vyasa, a major figure in Hinduism and one of the traditional authors of the Mahabharata, "yoga is samadhi." This is generally interpreted to mean that Samadhi is a state of complete control (samadhana) over the functions and distractions of consciousness.

In practice Samadhi is said to be the state of being aware of one's Existence without thinking, in a state of undifferentiated "Beingness." Three intensities (depths) of Samadhi are usually understood in Hinduism.

1. Laja Samadhi
2. Savikalpa Samadhi
3. Nirvikalpa Samadhi (or Sahaja Samadhi)

Laja Samadhi is a latent ("laja"), potential level of samadhi. It begins in deep meditation or trance-even with movement, such as dancing. This kind of samadhi is a state of joy, deep and general wellbeing, and peaceful meditation.

Savikalpa Samadhi refers to the initial temporary state of full-valued samadhi. The conscious mind is still active, as is the kalpa, meaning imagination. One should compare this meaning to that of sankalpa, which is "wish." Kalpa takes on a different, but related, meaning to sankalpa because one must use imagination or consciousness (kalpa) to envision a wish or desire (sankalpa). Conversely, vikalpa means "against imagination." At this final level of samadhi, the mind has become quiet and given up its desires and attendant. Vikalpa leads to the Truth, releasing one from any binds of mind (which are mostly imaginations). In Savikalpa Samadhi, we get the taste of Bliss and Beingness, but are still attached to our erroneous identification with the body as well as to our numerous worldly attractions.

Nirvikalpa Samadhi is the end result. There are no more kalpas (imaginings, wishes or other products from work of the mind), because the mind is finally under control. Upon entering Nirvikalpa Samadhi, the differences we saw before have faded and we can see everything as one. In this condition nothing but pure Awareness remains and nothing is missing to take away from Wholeness and Perfection.

Entering samadhi in the beginning takes effort and holding on to a state of samadhi takes even more effort. The beginning stages of samadhi (Laja and Savikalpa Samadhi) are only temporary. By "effort" it is not meant that the mind has to work more. Instead, it means work to control the mind and release the self. Note that normal levels of meditation (mostly the lower levels) can be held automatically, as in "being in the state of meditation" rather than overtly "meditating." The ability to obtain positive results from meditation is much more difficult than simply meditating. It is recommended to find a qualified spiritual master (guru or yogi) who can teach a meditator about the workings of the mind.

Samadhi is the only stable unchanging reality; all else is ever-changing and does not bring everlasting peace or happiness.

Staying in Nirvikalpa Samadhi is effortless but even from this condition one must eventually return to ego-consciousness. Otherwise, this highest level of Samadhi leads to Nirvana, which means total Unity and the logical end of individual identity (and also death of the body). However, it is entirely possible to stay in Nirvikalpa Samadhi and yet be fully functional in this world. This condition is known as Sahaja Nirvikalpa Samadhi or Sahaj Samadhi (sahaja means "spontaneous" in Sanskrit). Only the truly Enlightened (Satguru) can be and remain spontaneously free.

In Nirvikalpa Samadhi, all attachment to the material world and all karma is dissolved. All awareness is withdrawn step by step from the physical, astral and causal bodies until self-realization or oneness with the soul is achieved. During this process, breathing ceases and the heart stops beating.

Aware and fully conscious oneness with soul is then achieved in a most loving way, and all cells of the physical body are flooded with the Ocean of Divine Love and Divine Bliss for any period of duration-hours, days, weeks, until the individual shifts his awareness from the soul back to the physical body. Being fully functional in this world, his awareness stays in connection with the Divine. But some "strange" conditions accompany this state-better health (the body is sustained by Divine Grace), better feelings (even for other people who may contact the body which the enlightened soul has reidentified with) and various miraculous happenings may occur in connection with the Enlightened one.

Mahasamadhi (literally great samadhi) is the Hindi term for a realized yogi's conscious departure from the physical body at death. Which is also known as Nirvana (see above).

Mahasamadhi is the final conscious exit from the physical body. Every infinitesimal piece of attachment or karma is completely surrendered unto God and dissolved into the Divine Ocean of Love. The individual transcends to worlds beyond karma and returns to God, merging into transcendental Bliss.

Samadhi in Bhakti

The Vaishnava Bhakti Schools of Yoga define Samadhi as "complete absorption into the object of one's love (Krishna)." Rather than thinking of "nothing," true samadhi is said to be achieved only when one has pure, unmotivated love of God. Thus samadhi can be entered into through meditation on the personal form of God, even while performing daily activities a practitioner can strive for full samadhi.

"Anyone who is thinking of Krishna always within himself, he is first-class yogi." If you want perfection in yoga system, don't be satisfied only by practising a course of asana. You have to go further. Actually, the perfection of yoga system means when you are in samadhi, always thinking of the Vishnu form of the Lord within your heart, without being disturbed... Controlling all the senses and the mind. You have to control the mind, control the senses, and concentrate everything on the form of Vishnu. That is called perfection of yoga"-A. C. Bhaktivedanta Swami Prabhupada

"Meditation means to absorb your mind in the Supreme Personality of Godhead. That is meditation, real meditation. In all the standard scriptures and in yoga practice formula, the whole aim is to concentrate one's mind in the Supreme Personality of Godhead. That is called samadhi, samadhi, ecstasy. So that ecstasy is immediately brought by this chanting process. You begin chanting and hear for the few seconds or few minutes: you immediately become on the platform of ecstasy."-A. C. Bhaktivedanta Swami Prabhupada

Samadhi, a Description

In his book Autobiography of a Yogi, Paramahansa Yogananda, a reputed modern-day spiritual saint of India and teacher of Kriya Yoga, gives this stirring description of Samadhi consciousness:

My body became immovably rooted; breath was drawn out of my lungs as if by some huge magnet. Soul and mind instantly lost their physical bondage, and streamed out like a fluid piercing light from my every pore. The flesh was as though dead, yet in my intense awareness I knew that never before had I been fully alive. My sense of identity was no longer narrowly confined to a body, but embraced the circumambient atoms. People on distant streets seemed to be moving gently over my own remote periphery. The roots of plants and trees appeared through a dim transparency of the soil; I discerned the inward flow of their sap.

The whole vicinity lay bare before me. My ordinary frontal vision was now changed to a vast spherical sight, simultaneously all perceptive. Through the back of my head I saw men strolling far down Rai Ghat Road, and noticed also a white cow who was leisurely approaching. When she reached the space in front of the open ashram gate, I observed her with my two physical eyes. As she passed by, behind the brick wall, I saw her clearly still. All objects within my panoramic gaze trembled and vibrated like quick motion pictures. My body, Master's, the pillared courtyard, the furniture and floor, the trees and sunshine, occasionally became violently agitated, until all melted into a luminescent sea; even as sugar crystals, thrown into a glass of water, dissolve after being shaken. The unifying light alternated with materialisations of form, the metamorphoses revealing the law of cause and effect in creation.

An oceanic joy broke upon calm endless shores of my soul. The Spirit of God, I realized, is exhaustless Bliss; His body is countless tissues of light. A swelling glory within me began to envelop towns, continents, the earth, solar and stellar systems, tenuous nebulae, and floating universes. The entire cosmos, gently luminous, like a city seen afar at night, glimmered within the infinitude of my being. The sharply etched global outlines faded somewhat at the farthest edges; there I could see a mellow radiance, ever undiminished. It was indescribably subtle; the planetary pictures were formed of a grosser light.

The divine dispersion of rays poured from an Eternal Source, blazing into galaxies, transfigured with ineffable auras. Again and again I saw the creative beams condense into constellations, then resolve into sheets of transparent flame. By rhythmic reversion, sextillion worlds passed into diaphanous luster; fire became firmament.

I cognized the center of the empyrean as a point of intuitive perception in my heart. Irradiating splendour issued from my nucleus to every part of the universal structure. Blissful amrita, the nectar of immortality, pulsed through me with a quicksilver-like fluidity. The creative voice of God I heard resounding as Aum, the vibration of the Cosmic Motor.

Suddenly the breath returned to my lungs. With a disappointment almost unbearable, I realized that my infinite immensity was lost. Once more I was limited to the humiliating cage of a body, not easily accommodative to the Spirit. Like a prodigal child, I had run away from my macrocosmic home and imprisoned myself in a narrow microcosm.

Samadhi as Leaving the Body

Advanced yogis have been said to consciously leave (or disidentify with) their bodies as a vital step in the attainment of this final samadhi, or soul-liberation. It is at this time that the soul knows a complete and unbroken union with the Heavenly Godhead, and, being free from the limitations of the body, merges effortlessly into the transcendent amrita of Divine Bliss. It is said that sometimes the yogi leaves the body and returns. According to Meher Baba, Jesus entered into nirvikalpa samadhi at the time of his crucifixion.

Samadhi in Buddhism

Samadhi, or concentration of the mind (one-pointedness of mind, cittassa-ekaggata), is the third division of the Eightfold Path of the Buddha's teaching: panna (wisdom), sila (conduct), samadhi (concentration). It developed by samatha meditation. It has been taught by the Buddha using 40 different objects of meditation, according to the Visuddhimagga, an ancient commentarial text. These objects include the breath (anapanasati meditation), loving kindness (metta meditation), various colours, earth, fire, etc. (kasina meditation). Upon development of samadhi, one's mind becomes temporary purified of defilements, calm, tranquil, and luminous. Once the meditator achieves a strong and powerful concentration, his mind is ready to penetrate and see into the ultimate nature of reality, eventually obtaining release from all suffering.

Important components of Buddhist meditation, frequently discussed (1, 2) by the Buddha, are the successively higher meditative states known as the four jhanas which in the language of the eight-fold path, is "right concentration". Right concentration has also been defined as concentration arising due to the previous 7 steps of the noble eightfold path in the Mahacattsarika sutta/MN.

Four developments of samadhi are mentioned in the Pali Canon:

1) Jhana
2) Increased alertness
3) Insight into the true nature of phenomena (knowledge and vision)
4) Final liberation

There are different types of samadhi mentioned as well:

1) access concentration (upacara samadhi)
2) fixed concentration (appana samadhi)
3) momentary samadhi (khanikha samadhi)
4) "concentraion without interruption" (anantharika samadhi)
5) immeasurable concentration (appamana samadhi)

Not all types of samadhi are recommended either. Those which focus and multiply the Five Hindrances are not suitable for development.

The Buddhist suttas also mention that samadhi practitioners may develop supernormal powers (abhijna, also see siddhis), and list several that the Buddha developed, but warn that these should not be allowed to distract the practitioner from the larger goal of complete freedom from suffering.

The bliss of Samadhi is not the goal of Buddhism; but it remains an important tool in reaching the goal of enlightenment.

It has been said that Samatha/samadhi meditation and vipassana/insight meditation are the two wheels of the chariot of the noble eightfold path and the Buddha strongly recommended developing them both.

Analogous Concepts

According to the book "God Speaks" by Meher Baba, the Sufi words fana-fillah and baqa-billah are analogous to nirvikalpa samadhi and sahaj samadhi respectively. The Christian state of "receiving the Holy Spirit" could also be viewed as analogous to laja samadhi. This is also similar to the Don Juan concept of "stopping the world" as described in the Carlos Castaneda books.

States of consciousness with some of the features of Samadhi are experienced by individuals with no religious or spiritual preparation or disposition. Such episodes occur spontaneously and appear to be triggered by physically or emotionally charged peak experiences such as in runner's high or orgasmic ecstasy, however even mundane activities such as revelling in a sunset, dancing or a hard day's work have, in rare instances, induced the entire range of Samadhi from Laja to Nirvikalpa.

The only distinction in these spontaneous secular samadhi from Vedic and Buddhist descriptions is that in the state of non-duality equivalent to Nirvikalpa, there is no record of any supernormal physical effects as purported in the literature such as the breath and heart-beat stopping or any degree of conscious control during the event. Also absent are siddhis-like special powers as an aftermath although virtually all experiencers report they became imbued with a holistic and compassionate world view and no longer feared death.

As consciousness is in a state of duality in Laja and Savikalpa Samadhi there are some similarities to those described in NDEs near death experiences or Bardo in which interactions with archetypal events or entities may occur. In contrast-once swept into Nirvikalpa Samadhi-consciousness is transformed to a state of absolute non-duality whose only manifestations are light, bliss and love.

CHAPTER

4

Pratyahara: The Forgotten Limb of Yoga Sutra

Yoga is a vast system of spiritual practices for inner growth. To this end, the classical yoga system incorporates eight limbs, each with its own place and function. Of these, pratyahara is probably the least known. How many people, even yoga teachers, can define pratyahara? Have you ever taken a class in pratyahara? Have you ever seen a book on pratyahara? Can you think of several important pratyahara techniques? Do you perform pratyahara as part of your yogic practices? Yet unless we understand pratyahara, we are missing an integral aspect of yoga without which the system cannot work.

The same as the fifth of the eight limbs, pratyahara occupies a central place. Some yogis include it among the outer aspects of yoga, others with the inner aspects. Both classifications are correct, for pratyahara is the key between the outer and inner aspects of yoga; it shows us how to move from one to the other. It is not possible to move directly from asana to meditation. This requires jumping from the body to the mind, forgetting what lies between. To make this transition, the breath and senses, which link the body and mind, must be brought under control and developed properly. This is where pranayama and pratyahara come in. With pranayama we control our vital energies and impulses and with pratyahara we gain mastery over the unruly senses – both prerequisites to successful meditation.

Pratyahara

The term pratyahara is composed of two Sanskrit words, prati and ahara. Ahara means "food," or "anything we take into ourselves from the outside." Prati is a preposition meaning "against" or "away." Pratyahara means literally "control of ahara," or "gaining mastery over external influences." It is compared to a turtle withdrawing its limbs into its shell – the turtle's shell is the mind and the senses are the limbs. The term is usually translated as "withdrawal from the senses," but much more is implied.

In yogic thought there are three levels of ahara, or food. The first is physical food that brings in the five elements necessary to nourish the body. The second is impressions, which bring in the subtle substances necessary to nourish the mind – the sensations of sound, touch, sight, taste, and smell. The third level of ahara is our associations, the people we hold at heart level who serve to nourish the soul and affect us with the gunas of sattva, rajas, and tamas. Pratyahara is twofold. It involves withdrawal from wrong food, wrong impressions and wrong associations, while simultaneously opening up to right food, right impressions and right associations. We cannot control our mental impressions without right diet and right relationship, but pratyahara's primary importance lies in control of sensory impressions which frees the mind to move within.

By withdrawing our awareness from negative impressions, pratyahara strengthens the mind's powers of immunity. Just as a healthy body can resists toxins and pathogens, a healthy mind can ward off the negative sensory influences around it. If you are easily disturbed by the noise and turmoil of the environment around you, practice pratyahara. Without it, you will not be able to meditate. There are four main forms of pratyahara: indriya-pratyahara – control of the senses; prana- pratyahara – control of prana; karma-pratyahara – control of action; and mano-pratyahara – withdrawal of mind from the senses. Each has its special theniques.

Control of the Senses (Indriya-pratyahara)

Indriya-pratyahara, or control of the senses, is the most important form of pratyahara, although this is not something that we like to hear about in our mass media-oriented culture. Most of us suffer from sensory overload, the result of constant bombardment from television, radio, computers, newspapers, magazines, books – you name it. Our commercial society functions by stimulating our interest through the senses. We are constantly confronted with bright colors, loud noises and dramatic sensations. We have been raised on every sort of sensory indulgence; it is the main form of entertainment in our society.

The trouble is that the senses, like untrained children, have their own will, which is largely instinctual in nature. They tell the mind what to do. If we don't discipline them, they dominate us with their endless demands. We are so accustomed to ongoing sensory activity that we don't know how to keep our minds quiet; we have become hostages of the world of the senses and its allurements. We run after what is appealing to the senses and forget the higher goals of life. For this reason, pratyahara is probably the most important limb of yoga for people today.

The old saying "the spirit is willing but the flesh is weak" applies to those of us who have not learned how to properly control our senses. Indriya-pratyahara gives us the tools to strengthen the spirit and reduce its dependency on the body. Such control is not suppression (which causes eventual revolt), but proper coordination and motivation.

Right Intake of Impressions

Pratyahara centers on the right intake of impressions. Most of us are careful about the food we eat and the company we keep, but we may not exercise the same discrimination about the impressions we take in from the senses. We accept impressions via the mass media that we would never allow in our personal lives. We let people into our houses through television and movies that we would never allow into our homes in real life! What kind of impressions do we take in every day? Can we expect that they will not have an effect on us? Strong sensations dull the mind, and a dull mind makes us act in ways that are insensitive, careless, or even violent.

According to Ayurveda, sensory impressions are the main food for the mind. The background of our mental field consists of our predominant sensory impressions. We see this when our mind reverts to the impressions of the last song we heard or the last movie we saw. Just as junk food makes the body toxic, junk impressions make the mind toxic. Junk food requires a lot of salt, sugar, or spices to make it palatable because it is largely dead food; similarly junk impressions require powerful dramatic impressions – sex and violence – to make us feel that they are real, because they are actually just colors projected on a screen.

We cannot ignore the role sensory impressions play in making us who we are, for they build up the subconscious and strengthen the tendencies latent within it. Trying to meditate without controlling our impressions pits our subconscious against us and prevents the development of inner peace and clarity.

Sensory Withdrawal

Providentially we are not helpless before the barrage of sensory impressions. Pratyahara provides us many tools for managing them properly. Perhaps the simplest way to control our impressions is simply to cut them off, to spend some time apart from all sensory inputs. Just as the body benefits by fasting from food, so the mind benefits by fasting from impressions. This can be as simple as sitting to meditate with our eyes closed or taking a retreat somewhere free from the normal sensory bombardments, like at a mountain cabin. Also a "media fast," abstaining from television, radio, etc. can be a good practice to cleanse and rejuvenate the mind.

Yoni mudra is one of the most essential pratyahara techniques for closing the senses. It involves using the fingers to block the sensory openings in the head – the eyes, ears, nostrils, and mouth – and allowing the attention and energy to move within. It is done for short periods of time when our prana is energized, such as immediately after practicing pranayama. (Naturally we should avoid closing the mouth and nose to the point at which we starve ourselves of oxygen.)

One more way of sense withdrawal is to keep our sense organs open but withdraw our attention from them. In this way we cease taking in impressions without actually closing off our sense organs. The most common method,shambhavi mudra, consists of sitting with the eyes open while directing the attention within, a technique used in several Buddhist systems of meditation as well. This redirection of the senses inward can be done with the other senses as well, particularly with the sense of hearing. It helps us control our mind even when the senses are functioning, as they are during the normal course of the day.

Focusing on Uniform Impressions

A different way to cleanse the mind and control the senses is to put our attention on a source of uniform impressions, such as gazing at the ocean or the blue sky. Just as the digestive system gets short-circuited by irregular eating habits and contrary food qualities, our ability to digest impressions can be deranged by jarring or excessive impressions. And just as improving our digestion may require going on a mono-diet, like the ayurvedic use of rice and mung beans (kicharee), so our mental digestion may require a diet of natural but homogeneous impressions. This technique is often helpful after a period of fasting from impressions.

Creating Positive Impressions

Another means of controlling the senses is to create positive, natural impressions. There are a number of ways to do this: meditating upon aspects of nature such as trees, flowers, or rocks, as well as visiting temples or other places of pilgrimage which are repositories of positive impressions and thoughts. Positive impressions can also be created by using incense, flowers, ghee lamps, altars, statues, and other artifacts of devotional worship.

Creating Inner Impressions

An added sensory withdrawal technique is to focus the mind on inner impressions, thus removing attention from external impressions. We can create our own inner impressions through the imagination or we can contact the subtle senses that come into play when the physical senses are quiet.

Visualization is the simplest means of creating inner impressions. In fact, most yogic meditation practices begin with some type of visualization, such as "seeing" a deity, a guru, or a beautiful setting in nature. More elaborate visualizations involve imagining deities and their worlds, or mentally performing rituals, such as offering imaginary flowers or gems to imagined deities. The artist absorbed in an inner landscape or the musician creating music are also performing inner visualizations. These are all forms of pratyahara because they clear the mental field of external impressions and create a positive inner impression to serve as the foundation of meditation. Preliminary visualizations are helpful for most forms of meditation and can be integrated into other spiritual practices as well.

Laya Yoga is the yoga of the inner sound and light current, in which we focus on subtle senses to withdraw us from the gross senses. This withdrawal into inner sound and light is a means of transforming the mind and is another form of indriya-pratyahara.

INDISPENSABLE AIDS TO THE PRACTICE OF PRATYAHARA

Pratyahara is roughly translated as "withdrawal". Withdrawal, it has already been seen, is an indispensable prerequisite to concentration. If you want to centralise the mind, first of all, it has to be interiorised. Because, if the mind is completely externalised and scattered over many things in this outer world of names and forms and human affairs, how can the question of concentration arise in such a mind? It is totally unequipped for centralising or focussing. It is not even inside. It is scattered over the seen world which is hundred per cent Prakriti or Maya as long as we perceive it through the senses. But the same outer world is seen by the illumined Brahma Jnani as Parabrahman through his Sakshatkara Anubhava, and so he says,"Sarvam Khalvidam Brahma; Sarvam Vishnumayam Jagat". For him, there is no Prakriti at all; there is Parabrahman only. The whole of the external universe is nothing but Parabrahman for him. "Sarvam Sivamayam" he says, "Sarvam Khalvidam Brahma". And the scriptures go on to say that there is nothing else besides Brahman—Neha Nanasti Kinchana. But that is a question of Sakshatkara. Whereas, our approach to this whole human situation of bondage and suffering is from the point of view of the Mumukshu, a Jijnasu who is in Ajnana.

A Word of Caution

The Mumukshu is not a liberated soul or a Jivanmukta Purusha. He is only a struggling soul, caught in the net of the bondage of Raga-Dvesha, of Asha-Trishna. So, we cannot apply the Sakshatkara principle to the actual situation of the Jivatma. And we cannot say that there is no Prakriti. We have to very much accept Prakriti. One little sight, one little sound upsets us, makes us completely forget our Self our real Svarupa, our Purushahood and makes us completely enslaved by passion, anger, greed, hatred, anxiety, fear, depression and dejection. We are subject to so many mental modifications, Chitta-Vrittis. So, in this situation, we cannot ride the high horse of Brahma-Jnana or Jivanmuktahood. We cannot truthfully say, "I am transcendental Purusha or Atman". We may practise saying it for the purpose of ultimate realisation. Such practice is called Brahma-Abhyasa Brahma-Chintana.

We may practise affirming our real nature and asserting it. But on the practical side, we have to behave with caution and commonsense. We cannot foolishly run into situations which will make us turn a somersault and have a terrible fall and weep. We have to be very, very careful in going about in our Vyavahara, because we are still very much in the grip of the original self-forgetfulness or non-awareness. We are very much in the grip of delusion, of Maya. So, Gurudev used to say, "It is all right to say that Brahman is beyond time, space and causation. There is no world for the Brahma-Jnanis. It is all right for them to say, 'I am Brahman; I am Jnana-Svarupa'. But, so far as you are concerned, if someone calls you a fool, you are immediately thrown into a violent temper, you are ready to quarrel with him, you are ready to fight, even to raise your fist. Let alone that, supposing you go and stand before some person and he is occupied with some other work, and does not pay attention to you, you feel very humiliated. You feel insulted. You will begin to think, 'Oh! This man is treating me like this'. So, let alone someone doing some harm to you, if someone fails to do something which you are expecting him to do, you feel very insulted. You salute someone and he does not return it, because he did not notice it perhaps, but you feel very bothered. Your whole mental mood changes.

It is all fine for you to say that there is no world in the three periods of time, but if you find that someone has forgotten to put salt in your Dal, immediately you cannot eat your food; you become upset. You say, 'What is this? You have not put salt'. Supposing someone gives you tea without sugar, your Brahmanhood is nowhere. You immediately become upset in the absence of sugar in your tea. You do not drink it as it is. You will demand sugar and ask for it and complain, 'No sugar has been put in my tea, no salt has been put in my Dal'. So, do not imagine things. Try to know where you are and start your Sadhana from that place". Gurudev used to say all this. You are surrounded by Prakriti; you are surrounded by various manifestations of Prakriti. And so the mind is externalised and scattered amongst the various names and forms and objects, and human situations and affairs, which constitute Prakriti. It is thus in a state of involvement with external Prakriti in all its various forms. And this situation is the very antithesis of the ultimate Yogic state that you are trying to reach.

Pratyahara—Start of the Return Journey to the Absolute

The metaphysical thesis and the philosophical background of Patanjali's Yoga Darshana says that you have to separate yourself completely from Prakriti and once again regain your splendid isolation as the independent Purusha, untouched by Prakriti and beyond all afflictions, supreme and in a state of perfection. Now you are involved in Prakriti; your mind is externalised, scattered amidst the various objects and experiences and affairs that constitute Prakriti. And there is the other experience awaiting you towards which you have to work, slowly and diligently, perseveringly. Your present situation and the situation you are aiming at are two extremes and therefore the need for Pratyahara. There is the need to practise Pratyahara.

If you want to transform your present situation which is the very opposite or contradiction of the ultimate state you are trying to reach through Samadhi and superconsciousness, you have to make a start somewhere. And so, the very commencement of the metaphysical transformation you are aiming to bring about is Pratyahara. In the Kathopanishad, this deplorable state of man is clearly mentioned when Yama tries to make Nachiketas understand that Brahma, the Creator, made the mind outgoing at the very time of creation. So, by its very innate tendencies, the mind is outgoing, because Rajo-Guna is present in it in considerable measure. Therefore, the Jivatma beholds only the outer universe and not the inner Self; and beholding only the outer universe, the Jivatma is subject to change, decay, modification and destruction. The

Jivatma finds no happiness; he weeps. And once a person recognises the situation, the cause of one's suffering, the cause of one's weeping, the cause of one's disappointment and frustration in trying to get happiness out of the external universe, the cause of one's disillusionment, once a person realises the situation he is in, if he has got real stuff in him, he makes up his mind about it all. "No, no" he says, "Happiness does not lie outside. I have made a great mistake, I have committed a great blunder. I shall reverse this state of affairs". Thus making a firm Sankalpa and determination, that exceptional being, that exceptional person, tries to reverse this process by making the mind go inward, by closing the doors of the senses, because he aspires to find true happiness, and he has understood now through Sruti-Vakya, Apta-Vakya and his own experience that real happiness and satisfaction is found in the Atman and not in the outer world of change and modification and decay. So he turns the gaze away from the outside and directs the vision inside. This is Pratyahara—turning the gaze away from the external and directing it towards the inner Self.

Some rare exceptional person, with stuff, with determination, with courage of conviction, with firm faith in the scriptures, in the words of the Guru, in the words of the elders, he it is that turns his gaze within. He turns his gaze within. Why? Because he desires to attain the indwelling Self. The rest of the masses, the majority of people that is, the great flock, they see only the external universe, they do nothing to change the situation; they do nothing to reverse the natural tendency of the mind. They allow it to flow through the senses towards the objective universe because they think that the objective universe is the only reality that exists.

There is no other Reality. For them, seeing is believing. What they perceive through the five senses, that is all there is. There is nothing else beyond. They cannot conceive of anything else beyond. So, foolishly thinking in this irrational short-sighted way, like children lacking proper vision and higher understanding, they make their life an entire affair of allowing their mind to flow through the senses and perceive only the external objects, and thus allowing, they get caught in the widespread net of Maya. And they come again and again into this world. There is no end to their wheel of birth and death. "Punarapi Jananam Punarapi Maranam Punarapi Jananee Jatare Sayanam". There is no end to this wheel. Again and again they go and come back, and weep and wail and laugh, and again go and come back. This ever-recurring wheel of death and rebirth, and death and rebirth, goes on for those small-minded ones, lacking understanding, thinking like children. Instead of thinking and acting like mature wise people, they think like children. So they come again and again into this world. Whereas, the Mumukshu is a Dheera, the Jijnasu is a Dheera, like Markandeya, like Nachiketas, like Dhruva, like Prahlada, Satyakama and Svetaketu.

They are Dheeras; they are people with the exceptional stuff. They have got inner strength, courage to follow their beliefs, and faith, and so they make all the effort that is necessary and turn the gaze away. They reverse the process of the natural tendency of the mind and try to take it inward towards the Eka or the One, instead of towards the Aneka or the many that lie outside. They try to take the mind towards the Sattva instead of towards the Nama-Rupa. They try to take the mind towards the Nitya instead of towards the Anitya. That is Pratyahara. And, from the purely psychological point of view, the purely scientific point of view, as a technique, you cannot do Dharana unless you have got Pratyahara. Pratyahara is an Abhyasa or a technique or a process that is indispensable if you have to carry out Dharana. If you must concentrate the mind, first of all the mind must be brought in, the mind must be made to come together; it must be turned inward. And this needs also sense-control. Unless you have got sense-control, you cannot do Pratyahara. If the senses are turbulent and always bounding towards the Vishaya-Vastu or the worldly objects, you cannot do Pratyahara. So, it requires Brahmacharya to do Pratyahara successfully.

Brahmacharya and Pratyahara

Brahmacharya means that sample of conduct, that lifestyle, which leads to ultimate Brahma-Jnana. Thus, Brahmacharya is a comprehensive term. That is why Patanjali has laid it down in his Niyama. Brahmacharya means self-control. Tapasya includes self-control. Therefore arises the necessity of Tapasya in relation to Pratyahara, of Brahmacharya in relation to Pratyahara. If you have no self-control and self-restraint, you cannot have Pratyahara. The mind will continue to be bothered by the uncontrolled and turbulent senses.

The senses have to be kept in check. The senses have to be disciplined. The senses have to be trained, have to be subdued; and consequently, Yama and Niyama are to be practiced throughout the entire course of your Yogic ascent right up to the point of Samadhi. Or else, if you do not keep up Yama and Niyama always with you, even after attaining the state of Dhyana, you can have a downfall. Even a Yogi can have a great downfall. So, you can never underestimate the importance of Yama and Niyama. You can never understate the need to keep them along with you right up till the last stages of the Yogic ascent.

Vairagya and Pratyahara

Secondly, if Pratyahara is to be successful, you must have Vairagya. What is it that drives the mind outside seeking sense sensual enjoyment and satisfaction? What is it that drives the mind outside? It is desire. It is Asha and Trishna. It is the thirst for sense enjoyment. It is Raga. Unless you develop dispassion towards the external world, towards objective enjoyment and objective possessions, unless you say, "No, I do not want anything", you cannot engage in successful Pratyahara. And unless you practise Pratyahara, you cannot get established in Vairagya or dispassion. So they are both interdependent. Pratyahara helps in becoming more and better grounded in Vairagya. Vairagya helps in succeeding in the procedure of Pratyahara. Without Vairagya you cannot have Pratyahara and Pratyahara is necessary to become well established in Vairagya.

At this moment, ask yourself a question. Why is it that the Jivatma has so many desires, so many cravings? "I must enjoy this. I must possess this. I must come into contact with this." Why all this craving? Vedanta tells you that it is due to a basic Avichara, a basic lack of proper philosophical enquiry. You do not keep up this enquiry continuously—this enquiry into the real nature of things, this enquiry into the real nature of the so-called sensual enjoyment. If you make a right enquiry, philosophy will tell you that this is not enjoyment, but this is suffering. What you think to be happiness is actually suffering. It is the cause of further suffering. Because, you go towards pleasure and you become enslaved by it. You become addicted to it.

If you don't find it you suffer. Thus, what you think to be enjoyment is actually suffering. These enjoyments that come due to the contact between the senses and the respective sense-objects—they are a source of sorrow, a source of suffering. Now a little bit of enjoyment, but afterwards suffering. "Ye Hi Samsparsaja Bhoga Duhkha Yonaya Eva Te" Who says this? Lord Krishna Himself.

As a result there is no actual happiness here. Misery is mistaken for happiness; pain is mistaken for pleasure, because this happiness increases your craving. It makes it all the more. By satisfying your desire, you intensify your desire, and when you intensify your desire, it becomes a source of great agitation and mental restlessness. When there is Ashanti in the Manas, in the Chitta, how can there be happiness? Ashantasya Kutah Sukham? There cannot be real happiness where there is constant agitation, constant restlessness in the mind due to innumerable cravings and desires. They are all together and you do not realise it, because you do not carry on Vichara. Where there is proper Vichara and Viveka, Vairagya is possible. Where there is no Vichara and Viveka, Vairagya is not sustained, Vairagya is not Pucca, it is not ripe, and it is Kachcha.

Occasionally it will help you, and at other times, at the time of need, it will abandon you. Vairagya will vanish, and you will be foolish, and to use an English expression, you will find yourself in a soup. You will get into hot waters because of temporary abandonment of Vairagya. And you will commit some very foolish thing. Afterwards, Vairagya will come again. Then, you will remember Vairagya. Therefore they say that it is better to avoid getting into a wrong situation rather than get into a wrong situation, repent, open one's eyes, and afterwards try to correct one. Be wise. Arise, awake. Be wise. Understand that discrimination and enquiry are very, very important I addition to become established in Vairagya, by which alone successful and effective Pratyahara is possible.

Svadhyaya and Pratyahara

Also understand the importance of Svadhyaya to Pratyahara, because it is through Svadhyaya that the Yogi is able to keep his Vichara and Viveka fresh and alive or active. With daily Svadhyaya, you begin to get a deeper and deeper understanding into the genuine nature of the world and things. Svadhyaya carries you wisdom. Svadhyaya brings you awakening. Svadhyaya keeps your Vichara and Viveka keen and sharp. That is the value of Svadhyaya and that is the connection between Svadhyaya and Pratyahara. And thus, with the help of Brahmacharya, with the help of Tapascharya, with the help of Svadhyaya, if you have your senses under control, and if you keep your Viveka and Vichara keen and active, then gradually, becoming an Avruta-Chakshu Jijnasu, becoming endowed with an internalised gaze, with the mind turned away from the external outside, you are able to gradually prepare yourself for the higher stage of Dharana or concentration.

This withdrawal of Pratyahara should be supported by Brahmacharya, supported by Tapasya, supported by Svadhyaya, and supported by the Vichara and Viveka developed through Svadhyaya and it should be always bolstered by Vairagya. Vairagya is very important if you must successfully practise Pratyahara. In addition, in this process of Pratyahara, gradually you begin to progress and advance in keeping your mind always internalised, not moving towards the senses but moving towards the Self, the inner focal point within. And as you progress in this practice of Pratyahara, a stage comes when the senses gradually begin to change their nature, begin to give up their Vishayonmukha Svabhava, their innate tendency of always going towards the external objects, of always going towards their respective sense-objects.

That nature they gradually begin to give up, having understood through Viveka, through Vichara, through Svadhyaya, through Satsanga, the foolishness of moving towards the external objects, having understood that the external world is an empty chimera, that there is no pleasure there, that there is no happiness there, that there is only pain there. By going towards fire, you will only get burnt. A child is attracted towards the brightness, the brilliance, of fire. And if it touches the fire, it will get burnt. In the same way, the moth goes towards its destruction by plunging towards a bright flame. The Sadhaka begins to understand that, likewise, in the glittering external world, there lays only harm or injury, unhappiness, sorrow, lamentation.

Once this idea is definitely implanted in the mind, the senses come under the influence of this new knowledge. Formerly there was a situation when the mind was constantly being influenced by the senses, powered by the senses, dragged by the senses. And now, a certain change has come over the mind. The whole situation is now reversed. Now, the senses, instead of influencing the mind, become influenced by the mind, because the mind has become established in

Vichara and Viveka and Vairagya, and has become well-grounded in its new attitude to the external world. As a result it says, "No, my welfare does not lie there.

My happiness lies inside". The mind becomes well established. In this conviction and determines not to go outside but to go inside. What happens then? This new determination of the mind has its impact upon the senses, and in this new condition the mind begins to influence the senses. And the senses now decide: "No, we will not drag the leader. We will follow the leader. The mind is our leader. We will do as he says". So the senses stay put; they no longer bound towards the sense-objects, but they acquire a state of repose. They consent to stay where they are and they give up their old habitual, innate tendency of going outward. So, the senses attain a state of Dama. The senses become subdued, they become docile, and they decide to follow the mind. Therefore they also become internalized. They stay in their centers.

They do not bother the Yogi any more. They no longer present themselves as factors which distract the mind and agitate the mind. So, the problem gets overcome. In place of the mind being dragged out by the senses, the senses now consent to be brought inside by the mind. They follow the new tendencies of the awakened mind dominated by Vichara and Viveka, dominated by Vairagya, dominated by a higher discrimination. Such a situation becomes most suitable and helpful for the Yoga practitioner to take up the actual process of concentration or Dharana.

LIGHT ON DIFFERENT ASPECTS OF PRATYAHARA

As soon as you sit upon your Asana for doing your daily Dhyana, then it is that the mind begins to roam all over the place; then it is that the mind begins to go into various directions and think of numerous objects. And there you have to be firm. As and when the mind goes out towards external thoughts, you have to bring it back again and direct it towards the focal point of concentration, towards the object of meditation. This tug of war process—some-times swinging that way, sometimes swinging this way—will go on for some time and this process is part of the Abhyasa of Pratyahara. You try to bring the mind back, withdraw it from where it wants to go and taste. The mind usually goes to various objects which it wants to taste.

And you say 'No' and bring it back. So, this Abhyasa of Pratyahara may be practised as you are sitting in the meditation pose and trying to concentrate and the mind begins to wander. Actually, what happens? You are inside the room, inside closed doors, closed windows, with only the blank wall before you, and your eyes too are closed. You do not even see anything. Still, why should various thoughts come, of objects that are outside, which are not before you, which are out of sight? One would expect that the objects out of sight would be out of the mind also, but they are not. They are very much in the mind, they come up from within. Why? Because you have been constantly taking the impressions of those objects into your mind. You have been putting in Samskaras. So they are there. You have been creating impressions of the objective world within the mind. They have sunk to the bottom of the mind-lake.

And when you sit for meditation, they rise up. They may be remote impressions from memory or they may be the most recent impressions from the day's Vyavahara or activity. For example, if you sit for meditation in the evening, what all had been there before you that day till evening time can come up and bother you during your evening meditation. Or if you sit for morning meditation, you may start thinking about all the objects that are likely to be encountered during the day. "I have to do this, I have to do that, I have to meet this man, I have to go to that place"—all such thoughts may start coming. Because you have taken impressions of them. And how can you avoid taking these impressions? The moment you step out into the world, you are always surrounded by things, by sense-objects.

They come to you through all the five Indriyas—sight, smell, sound, taste, and touch—and they go inside. The instant you come out of your room, you are right in the midst of Nama-Rupa, right in the midst of variegated names and forms. It is precisely because of this that you must know how to practise Pratyahara even during Vyavahara, how to practise withdrawal even when you are right in the midst of lots of things and people and activities. That is to say, you must learn the art of being detached inwardly, the art of inner detachment even in the midst of activity. And you must learn the art how not to allow the external objects to go right deep into your consciousness even if they pass before your eyes like in a kaleidoscope or like on a cinema screen. The objects may present themselves to the eyes, and through the eyes they may be taken to the brain-centre inside. You cannot help seeing them. You may not deliberately want to look at them, but when they are before the eyes, you cannot help seeing them. You may not deliberately want to listen to something, but you cannot help hearing things anyway, because the ear catches sound, just as the eye catches sight. In this situation, what should you do? Detach the mind from the seeing centre, the hearing centre, the touching, smelling and tasting centres.

Separate the mind; let it have some other background. Let it have some other focal point, even in the midst of Vyavahar. That is why it is said that the Yogi should carry on unbroken God-thought. There must be a present of unbroken God-remembrance within himself, always, always...in the mind. If there is unbroken God-thought in the mind, that God-thought would form the permanent background for the mind. And the mind would recede into that background whenever it is detached from the external world. So, you must cultivate the habit of staying inward partially, even amidst your Vyavahara, not giving hundred per cent of the mind to external things and being completely overcome by sights and sounds, etc. You should study to give only a part of the mind to outer Vyavahara, merely that much of the mind as is completely necessary and necessary, keeping the rest in God-thought. Instead of blending the mind completely with sense-objects and becoming one with them, you must learn to give to the external things only as much of the mind as is necessary, keeping the rest of it inwardly detached. That is Pratyahara, as it should be practised even while you are in the midst of Vyavahara. Do not take in the impressions of the various perceptions too deeply into your mind. At the most, let the impressions touch the instruments of perception—ear, nose, eye, etc.—and from there let them be conveyed to the brain-centres of perception. Thus perceive them, but do not react to them. Let not the mind be too much concerned. Bring about a detachment of the mind from the perceiving centres in the brain. This is one aspect of Pratyahara.

There is one more aspect to Pratyahara. Supposing, before you know, the impression has already entered the mind. The mind has started to think about this impression. All right. Detach the ego from the mind. Separate your doer-ship. Say, "I am not seeing, I am not hearing. I am not interested in it. The mind has grasped it, true, but I am not the mind. I will step back and be a dispassionate, unaffected, unattached witness-consciousness. I have not taken the impression. My mind has taken it, my mind is thinking about it, but I will not identify myself with this line of thought". Thus asserting, you can bring about a withdrawal of the conscious "I" from the mind and its thoughts. Thus, disconnect your link with the mind. Do not say, "I am seeing, I am doing, I am thinking, I am feeling, I am hearing". No. Say, "I am neither thinker nor hearer nor seer. I am the witness-consciousness. These processes that go on, I only witness them. They will not affect me. I will not allow myself to be affected by them". In this way, bring about a severance of the connection between your ego-consciousness and your mind. That is also part of the

Abhyasa of Pratyahara in the midst of Vyavahara. There are some Yogis bring about a snapping of the link between them and the outer world, between them and the objects; they go away to Gangotri or they go away to some place where no one comes to them.

They keep alone by themselves. That is one technique of withdrawal—withdrawing oneself from the external objects. But that is not possible for all. You have to live and move among external objects. So, if you cannot break the link between the objective world of names and forms and yourself, at least snap the connection between the mind and the Indriyas or the perceiving centres in the brain. That is one successful step of withdrawal. Going deeper still, break the link between your ego-consciousness and whatever is put before the mind. Then, even if the mind has taken in some impressions or some thought-currents, you will stand apart from them; you will refuse to identify yourself with them. You will try to be Kevala Sakshi-Matra. This is the practice of actual Pratyahara or withdrawal. Even during the moments of actual activity and Vyavahara, in the midst of things, if this Abhyasa goes on, then the problem which arises when you actually sit upon the seat of meditation and try to withdraw the mind, that problem will be much lessened. The problem will be a great deal lighter, because you are already not allowing this problem to take root in the mind.

Perception is automatic and spontaneous. It cannot be prevented. If you go out, naturally the eye will see, the ear will hear, every sense will function in its natural condition as it is meant to function. But, if you cut off the link between the mind and the inner sense-centre, the outer sense may perceive the object and the inner sense may register it, but the mind will refuse to pay attention to it. And if somehow the mind gets involved in the perception unconsciously, then detach your ego from the mind and assert that you are only a witness, that the perception will not touch you, and that it has nothing to do with you.

The sense perceives and the mind is involved in it, but you will remain only a detached, unaffected, witness-consciousness. It can then have no impact upon you. It can then bring about no change in your consciousness. Your consciousness is established in its own essential nature which is non-duality, which is peace, which never changes. So, detach the real ego—not the false ego which is a part and parcel of the mind—from the mind and remain as the witness-consciousness. Now, it is the higher discriminating intellect that has succeeded in awakening the higher awareness, an awareness of the Reality, an awareness of your essential Self. That higher discriminating intellect counters the effect of the involvement of the mind. Mind is the emotive mind; mind is the desire nature. Mind is nothing but the spontaneous nature of emotion and desire. That may get involved due to being interested in the sense perception, but the discriminating intellect now ranges itself on the side of your essential nature and counters the involvement of the mind and says: "No, I refuse to get dragged into this. I refuse to associate myself with this present condition of the mind. I stand apart from it. I am only a witness of it". Thus saying, the intellect identifies itself with the pure consciousness which is unchanging and refuses to associate itself and identify itself with the mind and its present condition.

PRACTICE OF PRATYAHARA—AN EXERCISE AS WELL AS A PROCESS

Pratyahara, it may be noted, is both an Abhyasa in addition to a Prakriya. Abhyasa means a practice that you do at a given time, in a given place, in a particular Asana; and it is in the form of an exercise. And in the form of an exercise, it becomes a precious precursor to starting your meditation, because when you sit for meditation, your senses begin going outside. And in their wake, the mind begins thinking of objects. Thus, you have to withdraw the mind away from the senses. In that sense, Pratyahara is an Abhyasa. But in a more vital sense, it is a process. Pratyahara is not only a practice or an exercise, but it is also a process—a process that has to be constantly kept going throughout your wakeful hours of Vyavahara. Because, if you are trying to centre yourself in the inner Reality, in the Dhyana Lakshya or object of meditation, that effort is confined only to your hours of actual practice. And the rest of the time you allow the mind and the senses to go in the opposite direction towards the external things, towards the many things or the Aneka, towards the perception and enjoyment of sense-objects. So, what happens? Your Yoga practice will never succeed. Your inner Yoga practice can never succeed. It can succeed only if it has the full cooperation and support of the remaining part of your life, that is, your life outside the meditating hours, because you're Yoga Abhyasa has to be done within the broad framework of your normal life. Your normal life you cannot ignore. You cannot make it disappear. There is no magic wand to do that. Your normal life is there, very much there. Day after day, the Yogi has got to cope with a certain pattern of external life.

At this juncture we are talking of the vast majority of Yogis in the workaday world. We are not talking of the microscopic minority, the few who may have succeeded in completely isolating themselves from the rest of the world and who may be staying in a cave in Gomukh or Gangotri. Such Yogis are only a microscopic minority and their pattern of living has no relevance to reality, has no relevance to the rest of the people who are all striving upon the same path. Departure aside this minority, the vast majority of Yogis and practitioners has got a certain pattern of external life to deal with. They have got to cope up with it, and at the same time, they are authentic Yogis. They are as much genuine Yogis as the Yogis isolated in some remote seclusion, because their aspiration is as much real. Their desire for God and liberation is genuine. Even as the cave Yogi is trying to pursue his Sadhana in an extreme fashion, the generality of Yogis pursue their Sadhana as best as they can. Nevertheless, people belonging to either category are hundred per cent genuine, authentic Yogis.

At the present, in the context of the majority type of Yogis, Pratyahara cannot be an unhampered and undisturbed process of Abhyasa, completely cut off from the objective universe and all its distractions. In the case of the Yogi in isolation, there is not much of the objective universe there except his own body and the mountain and the rocks and Gangaji and the sky.

But the majority of the Yogis striving to lead a life of Yoga may be in a city-surrounding or a town-surrounding or in any normal surrounding with their own families to look after, business to attend to, or service to be done. In their case, the special Abhyasa or exercise will be a small part of Pratyahara.

They have to do their Yogabhyasa in the context of their social life, in the context of their professional activities, their home and family surroundings and environment.

Every one of them has his preoccupations with his family, with his children, with his wife, with his profession, business or service, with his social engagements. For Yogis of this group, then, Pratyahara will be extremely significant in its aspect as a continuing process throughout their waking hours, throughout their active hours, rather than in its aspect as a special exercise in the meditation chamber. For them, Pratyahara has to become a way of life. They have to live a life of Pratyahara. They have to practise Pratyahara in the midst of their daily activities at home, in society, in their specific field of professional life, in their specific field of service or business. In the Udyogic Kshetra, in the Samajik Kshetra, in the Parivarik Kshetra, in the Griha Kshetra—in all these places they have to practise Pratyahara.

And this is precisely one of the salient features of the Gita Yoga. "To be in the world and yet not to be in it". And, long,

long ago, when in his early days Mahatma Gandhi made a Gujarati translation of Srimad Bhagavad Gita, he gave that translation the name "Anasakti Yoga".

"Asakti" means attachment. "Anasakti" means detachment. Gandhiji called his Gita translation "Anasakti Yoga" or "The Yoga of Detachment"; and he said that this was the message of the Gita. In the midst of the world, be detached from the world, like the lotus in the lake, unaffected and uncontaminated by water. The lotus is in the water, but it does not become wet. Similarly, one should be in the world, but be unaffected by the world. In this way one should live. And this is the process of living a life established in Pratyahara. You have to practise this type of Pratyahara in the midst of activity so that outer perceptions do not have an ultimate impact upon you. You are in a crowd and yet you are alone. You are involved and occupied in various activities. Why? Because it is your duty.

It is your Kartavya Karma; it happens to be part of your Dharma. May be, you have to involve yourself in many things on account of your children, on account of your wife, on account of the marriage of your daughter, on account of trying to fix up your son in some job, on account of some litigation which has been forced upon you by your relatives or neighbours. There is no going out of all this. Yet, in the midst of it all, you know that you have nothing to do with it all. It is not because of your personal desire that you are involved in these things, it is not that all this Vyavahara has got some fascination or some attraction for you, but because they happen to be the immediate duties brought before you. You have no desire in the matter, but it happens to be your Kartavya Karma, it happens to be your Dharma as the head of the family. Wherever you may be placed, you have a certain duty to fulfil, a certain Dharma to discharge. In a particular location, in a particular context, you have a certain Dharma to fulfil. This is precisely what Krishna was trying to make Arjuna aware of on the battle field of Kurukshetra.

"Yogastha Kuru Karmani"—Essence of the Gita Teaching

Sri Krishna told: "Look here, Arjuna, whatever your personal sentiments may be, you are a prince of the Kshatriya race, of the warrior clan, whose Dharma is to defend the country and look after the welfare of the subjects and maintain law and order and Dharma. Here is absolute chaos. These unrighteous people have got the upper hand and they are bringing their unrighteous tyranny upon the people. The people are unhappy. Dharma is being completely destroyed. At the helm of affairs there is a complete absence of Dharma. So this is a Dharma-Yuddha, a righteous war. So, as a Kshatriya, as a prince, it is your duty to fight.

And, furthermore, on this first day of the War, you have taken over the task of leading your army as the Commander-in-Chief. So you must fight. It is your Dharma". So, Arjuna had this duty to do; it was facing him as his immediate duty also. Furthermore, he had assumed his duty, agreed to perform it, and come right upon the battle field, with the opposing army facing him there. In that particular context of his position as Commander-in-Chief of one of the two armies on the battle field, as prince of the Pandava race, this man's hundred per cent duty was to fulfil his particular role, to fulfil the Kartavya Karma which was facing him. It was his Dharma in that particular context to lead the army and try to see that the unrighteous Kauravas were overcome and defeated.

Subsequently, when Krishna told Arjuna that he must fight, what He meant was that Arjuna must do his duty—the duty which then faced him. The general notion of people that the Gita is a gospel of violence, a gospel of war, is a mistaken notion. It is a misconception. It betrays a complete failure to understand the central message of the Gita. Because the Gita happened to be delivered in a particular context, in the context of the battle field, the dramatic effect of it was heightened. Arjuna was told that even in the midst of the war, he was to be completely detached. He was to be established in God. He was to be rooted in God-remembrance. The Lord gave him this Sandesh: "Mamanusmara Yudhyacha. Remember Me constantly and fulfil your duty". When the Gitacharya, Lord Krishna, addressed these words to Arjuna by the word "Yudhyacha" He meant only, "Do your duty". And it just so happened that at that particular hour Arjuna's duty was to fight as a warrior in a righteous war. Be it noted that Krishna's emphasis was not so much on the word "Yudhyacha" as upon the word "Mamanusmara".

If the Gita had been preached to a Brahmin in a forest hermitage, this word "Yuddha" would never have got into the Gita. It would have taken a different terminology altogether. What the Lord meant to say was that even in the midst of the most intense and dynamically active field of human life, one should be in a state of Yoga inside—"Yogastha Kuru Karmani". The entire emphasis in the Gita is: "Wherever you may be, and whatever you may be doing you must be in a state of Yoga. You must be closely linked up with the Universal Soul. You must be closely linked up with the Divine, and thus linked up, you must perform your activities".

thus, it means that when this message, this teaching, this Yoga, that you must be linked up with the Divine and perform activities, that you must be grounded in God-remembrance and God-thought even while performing your activities, could be prescribed even in the tense circumstances of a battle field, then it goes without saying that it applies to all other fields of human activity. The most difficult field of human activity is naturally the field of battle, where the people clash and kill under the most violent, most dynamic and most complicated circumstances. And if Yoga can be practised there, then no one can give an excuse that he cannot practise Yoga because he is a business man or he is a somebody else.

If Lord Krishna had given His message in some other context, then the soldier of the battle field might have protested that the Upadesh or teaching could apply to anyone else, but not to him because he was in a very, very complicated and difficult field, namely, the life-and-death battle field. Evidently, the Lord deliberately chose the most difficult, the most complicated, the most active and most violent, and the most externalised field of activity that is ever possible for a human being to practise the Gita Yoga of inward living. If the Gita Yoga is possible in the midst of the clash and clang of weapons in a field of battle, then it is possible anywhere and everywhere. Then, no one can ever come forward and say, "No, it is not possible in my particular context, in my particular circumstance". So, once and for all, the possibility of anyone putting forward an excuse for not practising the Gita Yoga was effectively removed by the Lord when He chose the battle field to give His Upadesh to Arjuna.

It is in the above context that we must understand Pratyahara also. You must learn to be detached in the midst of activities. You must learn to be grounded in the inner background in the midst of outward activity or outer dynamism. And this process of Pratyahara is an indispensable necessity if you want to practise Yoga in daily life. If you want to practise Dharana, Dhyana and Samadhi in the context of a normal life lived in the world, the support of the process of Pratyahara in the midst of your normal activity becomes most significant and most important. Nay, it is indispensable. So, Pratyahara as a process has a greater importance to the Yogi in the normal context of worldly life than Pratyahara as a practice at a particular time just before meditation.

Indispensability of Vichara and Viveka for Successful Pratyahara Practice

At present, the moment you move towards the external scene, you are surrounded by external objects, and each external object has got its own fascination for you. Each external object has got its own attraction for your mind due to long association. And naturally, the moment you are amidst those objects, this attraction starts pulling you out, because the mind is constituted that way. Every object is found to be desirable for some purpose or the other. The fascination of Nama-Rupa to the Chitta is part of the function of Prakriti, because the whole of Prakriti is nothing but Maya, and Maya is full of this power of tremendous attraction to delude the Jiva.

Thus, if you have to keep up the process of Pratyahara during the hours of normal daily activity, you have to have the process of philosophical enquiry and discrimination constantly active. You must constantly exercise your faculty of discrimination to distinguish between what is real and what is unreal. This is what is known as Nitya-Anitya-Vastu-Viveka or Sat-Asat-Vastu-Viveka or Atma-Anatma-Vastu-Viveka.

You must also reason thus: "This object is attracting me; my mind is being pulled towards it. The senses are bounding towards it. Is it going to bring me any good? Out of this, can I achieve my welfare? Is it going to be conducive to my peace of mind? Will I get real happiness out of it? What is it going to give me?" This is Vichara. This is enquiry. You must tell your mind: "This object will give me only more confusion, more Trishna, more restlessness and agitation. Where there is desire, there is agitation, restlessness of the mind. The more I give in to it, the more the desire will intensify and multiply.

This is the Law. A desire that is around in the mind never subsides with the satisfaction of the same. On the contrary, satisfying the desire only makes the desire-fire to blaze up with renewed vigour, with redoubled vigour.

Desire is like a fire being fed with oblation—Ghee or oil. It will not receive the oblation and subside; on the contrary, it will blaze forth with redoubled vigour. Fulfilling the desire, surely, is not the way to overcome it. So I must renounce the desire, give up the desire. Rushing towards sense-objects will bring only ruin upon me. It will bring about greater restlessness, greater intensification of desire, and more agitation. No, I will not allow my mind to be dragged away by the senses towards these sense-objects". Such Vichara should be there, active Vichara or philosophical enquiry.

Upon the basis of what you have learnt from the scriptures, upon the basis of what your Guru has told you, upon the basis of what saints and sages have taught you as a result of their own experience of this world, this world is hollow, this world is only a Mriga-Marichika, a mirage in the desert. You will run towards it and you will perish. Nothing will come; there is no water there. Therefore, do not be deluded by the sense-objects. Move away from them; be a Master. In the light of your own life in this world, you yourself know what bitter experiences you have by rushing towards objects. "Once bitten, twice shy" they say. Once you have known the real nature of fire, will you again go towards fire? Like that, upon the basis of your vivid recollection of your own previous experiences, upon the basis of whatever knowledge you have gleaned from your study of the scriptures, upon the basis of what your Guru has told you, upon the basis of the teachings of the saints and sages, you must be ever alert and vigilant and keep your discrimination constantly active.

You must always do Vyavahara as a Viveki; then only you will be able to have Pratyahara in the midst of Vyavahara. If you want withdrawal and a state of detachment in the midst of active involvement in the objective universe, then this withdrawal is possible only if you constantly have this active philosophical enquiry into the illusory nature and the defective nature and the painful nature of sense-enjoyment. Wherever there is Vichara and Viveka, where there is such enquiry and such discrimination, then Pratyahara becomes progressive and successful. You can maintain Pratyahara in the midst of your activity. Then what happens? You come into contact with sense-objects, but they are never able to have their impact upon your inner consciousness. In your inner consciousness, you are always detached. The sense-objects may go only as far as the senses, they may go even as far as the inner centres of sense perception, but they will not be able to affect the mind, they will not be able to put the mind in a turmoil. They will not disturb your mind, much less your inner consciousness. Thus do you effectively succeed in preventing the external perceptions from making any impact upon your consciousness?

What does that mean again? It means that you no longer create any new Samskaras. You no longer create any new Vasanas for yourself. Otherwise, the whole life is nothing but the almost continuous loading of your Chitta with more Samskaras and more Vasanas. If you go and involve yourself completely with external activities and objects, due to desires, due to attractions which make you succumb because of a lack of enquiry and discrimination, every sense perception, every experience, every sense contact that you engage in creates a new Samskara and a new Vasana. This is an unending process and you will never be able to liberate yourself. Already, a load of previous Samskaras and Vasanas are playing enough havoc by raising Chitta Vrittis within the mind, and the moment you sit for meditation these buried Samskaras and Vasanas are constantly coming to the surface and creating Vrittis and various ideas in the mind.

That is sufficient. Sufficient unto the day is the evil thereof. Why should you make a bad situation worse by acquiring new Samskaras and Vasanas? You may ask: "How can I prevent doing it?" Because, the moment you go into the external world, new Samskaras and Vasanas are created. The way of preventing new Samskaras and Vasanas is to see that no ultimate impact is made upon the consciousness even though hundreds of perceptions and sense contacts take place. Pratyahara effects this. Pratyahara succeeds in checking the sense perceptions from affecting the mind and touching the consciousness. The mind just refuses to take them in. They come to the outer sense organ or sense instrument; they come to the sense centre in the brain; but when they try to get to the mind, the mind says, "No. I do not want these. I shall not take these things".

Rarė Pratyahara of the Byzantine Monks

Pratyahara, as we have seen already, has a number of specific phases. One is withdrawing the senses from the sense-objects. But it is possible only for a person isolated in seclusion—an Ekantavasi in complete seclusion. It is not probable for the vast majority of people. Bringing about a disconnection of the senses from the sense-objects, going away from all sense-objects, going into absolute seclusion or Ekantavas is positively not for the vast majority. But, for the few who manage it, there are no sense-objects, there is no sense world, there is no cinema, no radio, no T.V. There is no Gulab Jamun, Jhangri and Pakodi; there is no silk and gabardine and velvet. Nothing. They have only the jungle and the rock and the river. Some monks isolate themselves even today in the Christian monastic set-up, where, the moment they enter into a monastery and are ordained as monks, they become dead to the external world. Inside the monastery, there is no contact with the outside world at all. They cannot receive any mail, they cannot read any newspaper, they cannot read any book. They are absolutely dead to the world. Their monastic routine completely absorbs their entire attention day after day, month after month, year after year, until they die and are buried. And when they are buried, no identification mark is put upon their graves. Only a cross is put; we do not know whose body is lying underneath. No name, no date of birth or death. So, these monks, even when they are alive, are dead to the world, completely isolated. They do not know what goes on in the outside world.

Still today there are a certain set of monks living in a certain part of Greece who are still living in a state of time that existed more than a thousand years ago. They follow a certain time-schedule which is called the Byzantian Time, because they went into this area and settled down as monks in the time of the Byzantian Empire, and that Byzantian Time is about six to six and a half hours in advance of our time. When it is six or seven in the morning here, it is already noon or midday for them. So, their sunrise and day start at about 1-30 a.m. when their clock will show 6-30 a.m. So, they still live only according to their time. When it is 7-00 a.m. in our timepiece, it is already midday, past midday, for them. So, they live according to that time even today.

They belong to the Eastern Church, not the Western Church which has its allegiance to Rome, to the Vatican, to the Pope. They do not have any Pope. They are called the Eastern Church and they also call themselves the Orthodox Church. There are two groups—one belonging to Russia (the Russian Orthodox Church) and one belonging to Greece (the Greek Orthodox Church)—and they still maintain that old tradition. Generally, putting the two Orthodox Churches together, they call it the Eastern Church, as distinguished from the Western Church which is founded under the Pope in the Vatican. So, the Byzantine monks live a life totally oblivious of what goes on in the outside world. Many of the Byzantine monks in Greece, when I went there, did not know that two wars had taken place in 1914 and in 1948. They did not know who Hitler was and who Mussolini was; they did not know that World War II took place; they did not know that the atom bomb was dropped. They knew nothing. It was all news to them. They said, "We do not know what is going on in the outside world". And they do not know. They live there and they die there and very few of those people are left now, because new candidates and novitiates are not freely forthcoming now as in olden days to enter into that order of monastic life. And many of the big monasteries there are vacant. The place is called Mount Ethos. So, the Pratyahara life of those monks is something totally different. They have nothing to do with the external world.

Phases in the Process of Pratyahara

Although, for the vast majority of people who are in the outer context, Pratyahara becomes an indispensable requisite for entering into still deeper realms of the Yogic process, namely, concentration and meditation. In the lives of those who have isolated themselves, the question of further impact does not come, because they have no sense-objects around them. excluding, for those who have sense-objects around them, the first disengagement, namely, the withdrawal of the senses from the sense-objects is not possible. In their case, the senses are very much involved in the sense-objects and the withdrawal of the senses from the sense-objects is possible only at the time of their meditation. They go into their meditation room and close the door and then there are no sense-objects around then except the picture of their Ishta Devata, the picture of their Guru and their Japa Mala and Svadhyaya book. But, for the rest of the time, they are very much involved in the sense-objects and the first withdrawal is not possible.

The second withdrawal is the withdrawal of the sense centre or the perceiving centre in the brain from the actual sense. Let the eye look, let the eye see, but you do not involve yourself in this process of seeing. It is with reference to this withdrawal that both in the Upanishads and in the Gospel of Christ it is said that the ultimate realisation is possible only for that seeker who, even though having ears, does not hear, who even though having eyes, does not see. Such a seeker is blind even though having eyes. He is deaf even though having ears. That is the nature of the person who, even though he lives in the world, yet makes himself dead to the world, by refusing to allow his inner perception centres to cooperate with the outer organs of the senses. He succeeds in detaching the inner perceiving centres from the outer sense organs. But then, if this is not possible, or if somehow or the other an impression is made on the inner perceiving centre, then even as you are perceiving the object, let your mind say, "Yes, I see this, but I have nothing to do with it".

This last withdrawal involves detachment of the mind; it involves the severing of the mind's link with the process of perception, with the act of perception. In the beginning stages of Sadhana, the moment perception takes place, the mind becomes involved, because the mind is still in a state of desire and craving, in a state of Asha-Trishna. In that case, the "I" of the Sadhak which identifies itself with the awakened intellect, the Suddha Buddhi or the Jagrat Buddhi—which is now his best friend because it is Vichara-Yukta and Vivekatmaka—comes to his rescue. His Buddhi is now combined with active enquiry, combined with Viveka or discrimination. So, the ego-consciousness identifies itself with the awakened, discriminating and enquiring intellect and says, "I refuse to involve myself even in the mind.

I refuse to recognize myself with this state of the mind, with this condition of the mind, when it is perceiving this sense-object, when it is involved in this sense-object. I refuse to associate myself with this condition of the mind". So, the Sadhak who is endowed with this discriminating intellect now steps back and becomes only the detached witnessing consciousness. This is the withdrawal of the ego or the "I", the awakened "I", the discriminating "I", from the mental involvement in perception. So, one or the other of these phases of Pratyahara should always be present in your Antahkarana. The first one is not possible for the people who are involved in the world. The second, third and fourth phases should be actively exercised; they should be dynamically present in your Antahkarana at any time. Thus, Pratyahara is a continuous process. And for this withdrawal, constant exercise of enquiry and discrimination are indispensable. They are also part of it.

Pratyahara from the Scientific and the Metaphysical Angles

And this process of Pratyahara has a very significance in the overall practice of Raja Yoga and its special significance is twofold. One is the purely scientific significance—the significance of Pratyahara as an integral part or process of Raja Yoga as an exact science, a science of mind-discipline, a science of concentrating the scattered mind, a science of focussing the concentrated mind upon a single object, a science of practising this focussing in a continuous and unbroken manner. So, Pratyahara is a purely scientific process. So, from this scientific angle, Pratyahara becomes important and significant in the sense that unless you first of all withdraw the mind from being externalised, concentration is impossible. The question of concentration can never arise unless first of all the externalised mind is withdrawn. Only if you first succeed in withdrawing or internalising the externalised mind, only then can you try to bring about a centralisation of it inwardly. When the mind is not even inward, how can you centralise it? When the nature of the mind is completely extrovert and the mind is externalised, where comes the question of your trying to centralise it? First of all, bring it in. Then, within the context or framework of your interior, when the mind is still thinking of other objects, try to gather it together. Try to subdue its restless objectward motion or thought and try to bring it together. So, from the scientific point of view, Pratyahara becomes the indispensable qualification or prerequisite in order to be able to think of Dharana or concentration. No Pratyahara, no concentration. Unless you withdraw yourself, unless you withdraw your mind from the external things, you cannot have concentration. So, inner Yoga is impossible without first becoming well established in Pratyahara. Antaranga Yoga depends entirely upon successful practice of Pratyahara.

At present, leaving aside the scientific angle, from the metaphysical or philosophical angle also, you will find that Pratyahara becomes very, very significant. It becomes very, very significant in the context of the basic thesis, the prime thesis of Yoga. What is the prime thesis of Yoga? That all our woes, all our complications and all our problems have arisen due to the Purusha becoming involved in Prakriti. And the whole science of Yoga has been formulated in order to enable the Purusha to successfully disentangle himself from Prakriti and remain in his own pristine independent condition or native state.

And in the context of this prime thesis of the philosophy and metaphysics behind Yoga, you find now that Pratyahara plays a very significant part or forms a very significant phase in the Yogi's attempt to disengage and disentangle himself from his involvement in Prakriti. Now, what is the anatomy of your involvement in Prakriti? Through the channel of the senses the mind has been pulled out and embroiled or entangled in the objective universe. Why? Because the senses are turbulent, because the senses are outward-going, because the senses tend objectward, because the very nature of the senses is Vishayonmukha. And through the senses the mind is dragged out, and through the mind the Purusha gets completely involved in Prakriti, because the Purusha is in a state of total identification with the mind, which is one of its important Upadhis or limiting adjuncts. So, the Purusha weeps and wails, says, "Hai, hai", and is hopelessly imprisoned and entangled. And in this process of liberating the Purusha from Prakriti, Pratyahara takes on an added significance.

In the context of this philosophical background of the basic thesis of Raja Yoga, Pratyahara becomes an important phase of the Purusha—the Yogi—disentangling himself from involvement in outer nature or Prakriti, the world of names and forms, of Nama-Rupa, the world of Vishaya-Vastu, the world of Maya. In short, Pratyahara is the process of withdrawing yourself from Prakriti in the form of the external world of sense-objects. And so it has a very, very significant role, a specially meaningful role, in the overall process of the Purusha trying to disentangle himself from Prakriti once for all. So, that is the special place that Pratyahara occupies in the context of Dharana, Dhyana and Samadhi both in a scientific sense and also in relation to the ultimate liberation of the Purusha from Prakriti from the angle of the metaphysics and philosophy behind Raja Yoga.

CHAPTER

5

Samadhi Yoga: The Ultimate Yoga

All three Vedic Yogas all lead to Samadhi or the state of absorption with the indwelling Divinity. This Samadhi Yoga is symbolised by Soma, which is the Ananda or Amrita, the bliss or nectar of immortality. Letting the Soma or bliss energy flow is the basis of this, perhaps the highest of the Vedic Yogas. This requires an opening of all the nadis or channels of the subtle body, through which the Amrita or Soma can flow. This in turn requires proper development of all three Vedic Yogas.

THE DOCTRINES OF YOGA

What characterises Yoga is not only its practical side, but also its initiatory structure. One does not learn Yoga by oneself; the guidance of a master (guru) is necessary. Strictly speaking, all the other "systems of philosophy" as, in fact, all traditional disciplines or crafts are, in India, taught by masters and are thus initiations; for millenniums they have been transmitted orally, "from mouth to ear." But Yoga is even more markedly initiatory in character. For, as in other religious initiations, the yogin begins by forsaking the profane world (family, society) and, guided by his guru, applies himself to passing successively beyond the behaviour patterns and values proper to the human condition. When we shall have seen to what a degree the yogin attempts to dissociate himself from the profane condition, we shall understand that he dreams of "dying to this life." From the time of the

Upanishads India rejects the world as it is and devaluates life as it reveals itself to the eyes of the sage ephemeral, painful, illusory. Such a conception leads neither to nihilism nor to pessimism. This world is rejected, this life depreciated, because it is known that something else exists, beyond becoming, beyond temporality, beyond suffering. In religious terms, it could almost be said that India rejects the profane cosmos and profane life, because it thirsts for a sacred world and a sacred mode of being.

The Equation Pain-Existence

Yet this universal suffering does not lead to a "philosophy of pessimism." No Indian philosophy or gnosis falls into despair. On the contrary, the revelation of "pain" as the law of existence can be regarded as the conditio sine qua non for emancipation. Intrinsically, then, this universal suffering has a positive, stimulating value. It perpetually reminds the sage and the ascetic that but one way remains for him to attain to freedom and bliss withdrawal from the world, detachment from possessions and ambitions, radical isolation.

To "emancipate" oneself from suffering such is the goal of all Indian philosophies and all Indian mysticisms. Whether this deliverance is obtained directly through "knowledge" (according to the teaching of Vedanta and Samkhya, for example) or by means of techniques (as Yoga and the majority of Buddhist schools hold), the fact remains that no knowledge has any value if it does not seek the "salvation" of man.

The importance that all these Indian metaphysics, and even the ascetic technique and contemplative method that constitute Yoga, accord to "knowledge" is easily explained if we take into consideration the causes of human suffering. The wretchedness of human life is not owing to a divine punishment or to an original sin, but to ignorance. Not any and every kind of ignorance, but only ignorance of the true nature of Spirit, the ignorance that makes us confuse Spirit with our psychomental experience, that makes us attribute "qualities" and predicates to the eternal and autonomous principle that is Spirit in short, a metaphysical ignorance. Hence it is natural that it should be a metaphysical knowledge that supervenes to end this ignorance. This metaphysical knowledge leads the disciple to the threshold of illumination that is, to the true "Self." And it is this knowledge of one's Self not in the profane sense of the term, but in its ascetic and spiritual sense that is the end pursued by the majority of Indian speculative systems, though each of them indicates a different way of reaching it.

For Samkhya and Yoga the problem is clearly defined. Since suffering has its origin in ignorance of "Spirit" that is, in confusing "Spirit" with psychomental states emancipation can be obtained only if the confusion is abolished. The differences between Samkhya and Yoga on this point are insignificant. Only their methods differ: Samkhya seeks to obtain liberation solely by gnosis, whereas for Yoga an ascesis and a technique of meditation are indispensable. In both darshanas human suffering is rooted in illusion, for man believes that his psychomental life activity of the senses, feelings, thoughts, and volitions is identical with Spirit, with the Self. He thus confuses two wholly autonomous and opposed realities, between which there is no real connection but only an illusory relation, for psychomental experience does not belong to Spirit, it belongs to nature (prakriti); states of consciousness are the refined products of the same substance that is at the base of the physical world and the world of life. Between psychic states and inanimate objects or living beings, there are only differences of degree. But between psychic states and Spirit there is a difference of an ontological order; they belong to two different modes of being. "Liberation" occurs when one has understood this truth, and when the Spirit regains its original freedom. Thus, according to Samkhya, he who would gain emancipation must begin by thoroughly knowing the essence and the forms of nature (prakriti) and the laws that govern its evolution. For its part, Yoga also accepts this analysis of Substance, but finds value only in the practice of contemplation, which is alone capable of revealing the autonomy and omnipotence of Spirit experimentally.

The Self

Spirit ("soul") as a transcendent and autonomous principle is accepted by all Indian philosophies, except by the Buddhists and the materialists (the Lokayatas). But it is by entirely different approaches that the various darshanas seek to prove its existence and explain its essence. For the Nyaya school, soul-spirit is an entity without qualities, absolute, unknowing. Vedanta, on the contrary, defines the atman as being saccidananada (sat = being; cit = consciuosness, ananda = bliss) and regards Spirit as a unique, universal, and eternal reality, dramatically enmeshed in the temporal illusion of creation (maya). Samkhya and Yoga deny Spirit (purusha) any attribute and any relation; according to these two "philosophies," all that can be affirmed of purusha is that it is and that it knows (its knowing is, of course, the metaphysical knowledge that results from its contemplation of its own mode of being).

The Relation Spirit-Nature

If the Samkhya-Yoga philosophy explains neither the cause nor the origin of the strange association established between Spirit and experience, it nevertheless attempts to explain the nature of their association, to define the character of their mutual relations. They are not real relations, in the strict sense of the word relations such as exist, for example, between external objects and perceptions. Real relations, of course, imply change and plurality; now, these are modalities essentially opposed to the nature of Spirit.

"States of consciousness" are only products of prakriti and can have no kind of relation with Spirit the latter, by its very essence, being above all experience. However and for SamPhya and Yoga this is the key to the paradoxical situation the most subtle, most transparent part of mental life, that is, intelligence (buddhi) in its mode of pure luminosity (sattva), has a specific quality that of reflecting Spirit. Comprehension of the external world is possible only by virtue of this reflection of purusha in intelligence. But the Self is not corrupted by this reflection and does not lose its ontological modalities (impassibility, eternity, etc.). The Yoga-sutras (II, 20) say in substance: seeing (drashtri; *i.e.*, purusha) is absolute consciousness ("sight par excellence") and, while remaining pure, it knows cognitions (it "looks at the ideas that are presented to it").

Vyasa interprets: Spirit is reflected in intelligence (buddhi), but is neither like it nor different from it. It is not like intelligence because intelligence is modified by knowledge of objects, which knowledge is ever-changing whereas purusha commands uninterrupted knowledge, in some sort it is knowledge. On the other hand, purusha is not completely different from buddhi, for, although it is pure, it knows knowledge. Patanjali employs a different image to define the relationship between Spirit and intelligence: just as a flower is reflected in a crystal, intelligence reflects purusha. But only ignorance can attribute to the crystal the qualities of the flower (form, dimensions, colours). When the object (the flower) moves, its image moves in the crystal, though the latter remains motionless. It is an illusion to believe that Spirit is dynamic because mental experience is so. In reality, there is here only an illusory relation (upadhi) owing to a "sympathetic correspondence" (yogyata) between the Self and intelligence.

Pain exists only to the extent to which experience is referred to the human personality regarded as identical with purusha, with the Self. But since this relation is illusory, it can easily be abolished. When purusha is known, values are annulled; pain is no longer either pain or non-pain, but a simple fact; a fact that, while it preserves its sensory structure, loses its value, its meaning. This point should be thoroughly understood, for it is of capital importance in Samkhya and Yoga and, in our opinion, has not been sufficiently emphasized. In order to deliver us from suffering, Samkhya and Yoga deny suffering as such, thus doing away with all relation between suffering and the Self. From the moment we understand that the Self is free, eternal, and inactive, whatever happens to us sufferings, feelings, volitions, thoughts, and so on no longer belongs to us.

How is Liberation Possible?

Vedanta also criticizes the concept of the plurality of "selves" (purusha), as formulated by Samkhya and Yoga. For these two darshanas affirm that there are as many purushas as there are human beings. And each of these purushas is a monad, is completely isolated; for the Self can have no contact either with the world around it (derived from prakriti) or with other spirits. The cosmos, then, is peopled with these eternal, free, unmoving purushas monads between which no communication is possible. According to Vedanta, this conception is erroneous and the plurality of "selves" is an illusion. In any case, this is a tragic and paradoxical conception of Spirit, which is thus cut offnot only from the world of phenomena but also from other liberated "selves." Nevertheless, Samkhya and Yoga were obliged to postulate the multiplicity of purushas; for if there were but one Spirit, salvation would have been an infinitely simpler problem, the first man who should attain liberation would necessarily bring about that of the entire human race.

If there had been but one universal Spirit, the concomitant existence of "liberated spirits" and "bound spirits" would have been impossible. Nor indeed, in such a case, could death, life, difference of se+, diversity in action, etc., have coexisted. The paradox is obvious: this doctrine reduces the infinite variety of phenomena to a single principle, matter (prakriti); it sees the physical universe, life, and consciousness as derived from a single matrix and yet it postulates the plurality of spirits, although by their nature these are essentially identical. Thus it unites what would appear to be so different the physical, the biotic, and the mental and isolates what, especially in India, seems so unique and universal Spirit.

Vyasa [Yoga-sutras, I, I.] classifies the modalities of consciousness (or "mental planes," citta bhumi) as follows: (1) unstable (kshipta); (2) confused, obscure (mudha); (5) stable and unstable (vikshipta); (4) fixed on a single point (ekagra); (5) completely restrained (niruddha). Of these modalities, the first two are common to all men, for, from the Indian point of view, psychomental life is normally confused.

The third modality of consciousness, vikshipta, is obtained by fixing the mind "occasionally and provisionally," through the exercise of attention (for example, in an effort of memory or in connection with a mathematical problem, etc.); but it is transitory and is of no help towards liberation, since it was not obtained through Yoga. Only the last two of the modalities enumerated above are yogic "states" *i.e.,* brought on by ascesis and meditation.

The Subconscious

... at this point we can already recognise in Yoga a tendency that is specifically its own, and one that, therefore, we have not encountered in the Samkhya darshana. It is a tendency towards the concrete, towards the act, towards experimental verification. Even Patanjali's "classic" Yoga (and still more the other kinds of Yogas) accords the greatest importance to experience that is, to knowledge of the different states of consciousness. And there is nothing surprising in this, given the aim that Yoga in general pursues which is to rarefy, to dislocate, and, finally, to do away with these states of consciousness. This tendency towards concrete, experimental knowledge, in view of finally mastering that of which one has, so to speak, taken possession through knowing it, will be carried to its extreme by tantrism.

Long before psychoanalysis, Yoga showed the importance of the role played by the subconscious. Indeed, it is in the dynamism that characterises the unconscious that Yoga sees the most serious obstacle that the yogin has to overcome. This is because the latencies as if a strange impulse drove them to self-extinction want to emerge into the light, want, by actualising themselves, to become states of consciousness. The resistance that the subconscious opposes to every act of renunciation and asceticism, to every act that could result in the emancipation of the Self, is, as it were, the token of the fear that the subconscious feels at the mere idea that the mass of as yet unmanifested latencies could fail of their destiny, could be destroyed before having time to manifest and actualise themselves.

VEDIC INTEGRAL YOGA

These four Vedic Yogas together form an integral Yoga. They culminate in a complete or Purna Yoga. Generally the Purna Yoga relates to Indra and to Prana but in the expanded sense as the energy of consciousness and insight on all levels. However there is also a Purna Yoga of Agni called Vaishvanara Vidya (knowledge of the Cosmic Person), which proceeds through Self-enquiry. There is similarly a Purna Yoga of the Sun, particularly in the form of Vishnu or Savitar.

In this Purna Yoga the second world or the Atmosphere becomes the all world or the Cosmic Ocean, the ocean of the heart as the fourth world. This ocean is space and its waves are the wrolds. In the space within the heart is contained all the universe and the Supreme Self beyond all manifestation.

This leads to a slightly different formulation of the threefold Vedic Yoga:

1. Mantra Yoga - Earth - Body - Mother
2. Dhyana Yoga - Heaven - Head (Mind) - Father
3. Samadhi Yoga - Waters - Heart (Soul) - Child

The main form of Purna Yoga is meditation on the heart, which involves tracing the origin of speech, Prana and mind back to the Self in the heart, which is the main practice of Self-enquiry. This search is called gaveshana, or anveshana in Vedic texts. It is not done simply by repeating "Who am I?" but requires mantric and meditational control of speech, Prana and mind and an examination of all their movements in all states of consciousness as powers of the Atman.

The Vedic Yoga is vast and many sided. We have only outlined a few of its characteristic features. It has teachings which are appropriate for each individual and his or her level of development. It therefore has no mass teaching or standardised instruction. Each individual must be treated differently.

SAMADHI PADA I: CONTEMPLATION AND MEDITATION

Patanjali opens with a blessing for those seeking union (Yoga) with the supreme. Here the Seer/meditator/Yogi/self is equated to the soul and the concept of ego mind is introduced. The ego mind is composed of mind, intelligence and the ego which makes up the illusory self. When one learns to restrain or subjugate the ego mind then pure soul awareness becomes possible or knowledge of the true self becomes possible.

The illusory self is manifested as five fluctuations or fivefold movements: A blessing to those seeking instruction on joining (Yoga) with the Supreme Spirit.

Definition of Yoga

- Union (integration) of the self to the Supreme is the result of restraining fluctuations of the ego mind, controlling cognition and annihilating the ego.
- Then, at that time, the Soul (Seer) dwells in a state of radiance.

- At other times, the Seer, (Soul) identifies with the mind's behaviour of constant modification and fluctuation.

Obstacles to Union with the Supreme

- The mind modifications are composed of fivefold movements that are either afflicting or unafflicting, distressing or undistressing, pleasing or painful, troubling or untroubling, disturbing or undisturbing.
- The fivefold movements manifest as valid knowledge, perversion, imagination, dreamless sleep, and memory.
- Valid knowledge is achieved through direct perception, or the act of reasoning from factual knowledge and evidence, and from sacred texts or teachers knowledable of scripture and that which can be proven or verified.
- Perversion is actually unreal knowledge based on beholding not one's own form, but that which occupies illusion.
- Imagination is fanciful verbal knowledge invented in sequence that is devoid of substance, meaning or existence.
- Dreamless sleep is the means of going towards the true reliable abode of knowing the complete essence of one's eternal condition of non-existence, the thought-wave of feeling non-being. Dreamless sleep is the closest one comes to letting the self fall away.
- Memory is not allowing to slip away things experienced and is the recollection of perceptions, imaginations, thoughts, objects, senses and interactions with others.

Overcoming the Obstacles to Union

- The art of Yoga is the repeated practice of restraining the fivefold movements so one can detach from desires and achieve ultimate freedom.
- Practice is the continuous effort to achieve perfect restraint of these fivefold movements.

- To become firmly rooted with the Supreme requires that the practice be performed with zeal, dedication, and devotion continuously for a long time, without interruption.
- Listen and perceive this transmission of ancient testimony to achieving supreme joy and contentment through freedom from desires. To obtain union with the Supreme one must detach from desires and passions, for true understanding is accomplished by subjugating and controlling the fluctuations of the mind.
- The highest, most excellent supreme perception of pure soul awareness is achieved by trancending the three qualities of nature; (light, inertia and vibration).
- To actually distinguish true soul awareness one must grasp the four stages: It begins with self-analysis then personal insight trancending logic through meditation leading to blissful elation and finally universal consciousness.
- A lesser soul awareness is often achieved during meditation and practice that achieves a balance of mind with impressions registering below the threshold of consciousness. The intelligence is stilled but the impure awareness experiences visions or lucid dreams.
- This lesser state of soul awareness has its origins in the incorporeal realm of non-material existence which is the realm of spirit and law. Failure to trancend this state of being leads to isolation or a merging with nature.
- To continue progressing to pure soul awareness requires reverent faith, moral strength, keen memory and supreme devotion to profound meditation to achieve perfect absorption of thoughts and awareness of real knowledge acquired through intense contemplation.

- Pure soul awareness is near for those who continue to practice cheerfully and with intensity.
- Some proceed with mild effort, moderate effort or zealous effort and these levels of effort determine the speed one achieves pure soul awareness.

Surrender to God is the Ultimate Approach to Union

- The carnal mind can be transcended into pure soul awareness by profound prayer and meditation upon God and total surrender to God.
- God is the seat of Supreme Being, totally free from conflicts, unaffected by actions and untouched by cause and effect.
- God is the unsurpassed and unrivaled onesource of omniscent wisdom, transcendent, yet unfolds the entirety of omniscience, omnipotence and omnipresence.
- God is the unlimited, unbounded, undefined source of all knowledge and is the foremost absolute guru untouched by time.
- Aum (OM) is the sacred syllable signifying God and is the fulfillment of divinity and stands for the praise of the divine.
- The mantra Aum is to be repeated with reverent feeling with the aim of realising its identifying purpose,
- Thus removing the obstacles to acquiring the mastery of pure soul awareness.
- The obstacles to pure soul awareness are disease, procrastination, doubt, carelessness, laziness, attachment to sensual gratification, delusion, departing from practice and an unfocused mind.
- These obstacles exist at the same time with unhappiness, despair, unsteadiness of the body and irregular breathing which further scatters the mind and causes distractions.

- To prevent these obstacles, one should practice with single-mindedness the real state of truth so as to perceive the principal doctrine of essential nature thus revealing the very essence of pure soul awareness.
- But by being joyfull, glad, friendly, compassionate and merciful coupled with indifference to happiness and sorrow, virtue and vice, one will become infused with a graceful diffusion of pure soul awareness leading to a favorable disposition.

Techniques in Restraining the Fivefold Movements

- Helpful in restraining the fivefold movements is proper breath practice. This is done by steady slow exhalation followed by a pause before softly inhaling. This breath practice helps calm the mind and connect to soul awareness.
- Also progress can be advanced by contemplating an object with total absorption thus producing a mind state resembling the mind's foundational origins.
- Or, a tranquil state of mind can be the result of contemplating a luminous light of infinite brightness which is free from sorrow or grief.
- Pure soul awareness is achieved by unattachement to objects, desires and passions.
- In order to distinguish the gross from the eternal be cognizant of the three states of mind. The dreamless state of non-being, the dream state of delusion and the wakeful state of intelligent awareness.
- Mind dicipline can also be developed by meditation on a selected thing that is desireable and pleasing according to one's wishes or taste.

Benefits from Using the Techniques

- Mastery over passions and the fivefold movements brings the power over the infinitesimal to the Infinite.
- By trancending the three qualities of nature; (light,

inertia and vibration) and mastering the fivefold movements, the Yogi becomes like a flawless crystal gem exhibiting the characteristics of worthyness, wisdom, politeness, courtesy and distinquished nobleness. The Yogi is transformed into accepting that the knower, the instrument of knowing, and that which is known are not separate but are just modifications of the original form.

- At this stage the Yogi becomes totally engrossed in thoughtfull transformation as the word, its purpose, and the knowledge of the word become intermingled and mixed together such that the Yogi is trancendant of judgement. Instead the Yogi becomes the observer of reality.
- Now the Yogi is of the purest mind, cleansed of memory, devoid of the former nature, allowing the purest form of soul awareness to be as it is, unreflecting and unconsidered, without analysis or logic.

Subtle Techniques for Achieving Pure Soul Awareness

- In addition to contemplating objects and pleasing subjects, there are two other techniques of investigation. Both are related to the meditation of subtle things (such as ego, intelligence, time, space or causation) but one involves deliberate contemplation and the other is contemplation of the subtle without reflection or consideration. One involves logic and descrimination, the other intuition and a knowing transcendent of gross thought.
- Either technique of meditating on subtle things will lead to the ending of fluctuations revealing pure soul awareness, having no characteristic markings but only displaying its unmanifested form.
- Both techniques require profound meditation seeded by the core of being.
- But when the Yogi is skilled in profound reflection

without seeds, profound knowledge manifests as undisturbed pure flow of the union between the supreme awareness and individualised awareness, admitting maximum passage of clear bright light without diffusion or distortion, accompanied by serenity of disposition.

Achieving Ultimate Ttrancendent Wisdom

- The yogi's awareness now resides in insightful wisdom, full of truth and intellectual essence.
- This insightful wisdom has the special property of being beyond wisdom achieved by traditional means. This special wisdom is first hand intuitive knowledge of the Supreme and can not be gained by conjecture or inference.
- Now that the Yogi is born of supreme wisdom, previous formations of the mind become subliminal and the pure truth impedes future gross impressions.
- Even this new truth bearing light must be suppressed in order to achieve permanent seedless identity with the absolute supreme. By detaching from the supreme wisdom the Yogi drops away the remaining illusions of self and only the universal supreme soul blazes without form in pristine clarity.

SAMADHI IN YOGA

Samadhi is of two kinds *viz.*, Samprajnata and Asamprajnata. Samprajnata Samadhi is the first step. In this Samadhi, Samskaras are not destroyed. This is also known as Sabija Samadhi, because the seeds or the Samskaras are there. In this there is Alambana or support.

In Samprajnata Samadhi there are four varieties *viz.*, Savitarka, Savichara, Sananda and Asmita. All these will be explained in the subsequent Sutras. Samadhi can also be divided into two kinds, Sthula (gross) and Sukshma (subtle) that relates to Tanmatras and Indriyas. Samprajnata and

Asamprajnata Samadhis are termed as Savikalpa and Nirvikalpa Samadhi by Vedantins and Bhaktas. This Sutra refers actually to a series of meditations in an ascending order, first on the physical universe, then the subtle universe of potentials called Tanmatras, the cosmic complex known as space and time and cosmic Self sense leading to a bliss born of pure consciousness. Though the Sutra refers only to Vitarka, Vichara, Ananda and Asmita, they are further capable of categorisation as involved in space-time consciousness or not involved in space-time consciousness. These stages are intricate and cannot be understood by merely a study of books.

SAVITARKA SAMADHI

There the concentration in which the options of word, meaning and understanding are confused is called Savitarka Samadhi or the Samadhi with argumentation.

NOTES: If you concentrate and meditate on the gross objects, on their nature and in relation to time and space, it is Savitarka Samadhi (Samadhi with argumentation). It is Sthula Dhyana. You will get control over the object. You will acquire full knowledge of the object. You will get psychic powers (Siddhis).

The 'cow ' as a word, the 'cow' as an object and the 'cow' as an idea, though different from one another, are cognised as indistinct. You begin to analyse. The characteristics of the word are different; the characteristics of the idea are different; and the characteristics of the object are also different. Everything has a name which has some meaning. When the mind apprehends a word and meditates on its meaning and form as well as on the understanding of both, and thus lose itself in the thing completely, it is called Savitarka Samadhi. Sound causes vibration in the mind. It is carried through the external auditory meatus (external opening of the ear), through the auditory nerve to the auditory centre of the brain. Now a reaction takes place. The mind reacts. It understands the meaning of the sound. Now knowledge manifests. Now comes perception or cognition of the object. The mixture of these three, sound, meaning and knowledge constitute perception or cognition of an object. It is Savitarka Samadhi.

Savichara Samadhi

If you meditate on the subtle Tanmatras, on their nature and in relation to time and space, it is Savichara Samadhi (Samadhi with deliberation). This is Sukshma Dhyana. You will get knowledge of the Tanmatras. You will have great control over Tanmatras. Savitarka, Nirvitarka, Savichara and Nirvichara are called Grahya Samapatti.

Sananda Samadhi

If you give up the gross and the subtle elements, if you fix the Indriyas in their respective places and if you give up the gross and the subtle meditation, and if you meditate on the Sattvic mind itself, it is known as Sananda Samadhi. This is called Grahya Samapatti, cognition of the instrument of cognition.

Asmita Samadhi

When the Sattvic ego only remains during deep meditation, is called Asmita Samadhi. There is only Prajna of 'Aham-Tvam' in this Samadhi. The Yogi who has reached this stage is a Videha (without body). Prakriti- layas are those who in this state get themselves merged in nature. You will have to proceed further if you want Kaivalya. This is called as Grahitri Samapatti, cognition of the knower. Savitarka is gross Samadhi. Savichara is subtle Samadhi. Sananda is deep subtle Samadhi. Asmita is still more deep subtle Samadhi. These are all stages like the steps of an ascending stair-case.

Sabija Samadhi

These only, *viz.*, Savitarka, Savichara Sananda and Asmita are Sabija Samadhi or Samadhi with seed (Samskaras).

Samadhi

Samadhi is an intriguing mystery to the aspiring yogi who usually mistakes it for a psychic state productive of such physical phenomena as loss of outer consciousness, being without breath or heartbeat, and suchlike. Consequently many practice drastic and strenuous methods, especially breath control, attempting to stop their breath and heartbeat. And they are usually frustrated in their attempts and feel that they are not really making progress. One of the first saints I met was truly an earthly angel who by a single look could awaken the spiritual consciousness of others. He spontaneously healed souls and bodies. Yet, because of the influence of a guru he had studied with in his early years of spiritual quest, he often lamented to others: "I have not really gotten anywhere. In all these years I have not experienced the breathless state even once. So I have not even begun to progress." He was mistaking a physical condition for a spiritual one, as is common in both India and the West. So it is very important for us to understand what samadhi really is.

First of all, samadhi is our natural spiritual state. "The self is actionless and always in samadhi," says Shankara in his comments on the first Yoga Sutra. And: "As we have said, steadiness is samadhi. Rightly has the commentator [Vyasa] said that it is a quality of the mind in all the states."

Samadhi is the state of consciousness in which oneness with the object of concentration or meditation is experienced. In meditation it is the experience of oneness with the individual spirit (purusha) or the Supreme Spirit (Param Purusha). Swami Sivananda, in the Yoga Vedanta Dictionary, says: "Here the mind becomes identified with the object of meditation; the meditator and the meditated, thinker and thought become one in perfect absorption of the mind." From this we can see that samadhi is exclusively a state of awareness. Physical phenomena simply do not come into it, although certain conditions of the body may result as a side effect–especially in the case of beginners or those whose body and nervous system are not fully purified or controlled and so become overwhelmed and manifest various abnormal conditions. Because they are so dramatic, the states of breathlessness, absence of heartbeat, immobility or levitation are usually thought of in the West as being samadhi. As just stated, such states may accompany samadhi, but they are neither samadhi nor requisites or proofs of samadhi. "The fact of a person being in real samadhi is determined solely by the condition of his mind and not at all by the inertness of the physical body," asserts I.K. Taimni.

Patanjali discusses two forms of samadhi: samprajñata and asamprajñata. Sivananda defines them in this way: "Samprajñata samadhi: State of superconsciousness, with the triad of meditator, meditation and the meditated. Savikalpa samadhi." "Asamprajñata samadhi: Highest superconscious state where the mind and the ego-sense are completely annihilated." Both are produced by the practice of meditation–first samprajñata samadhi and then asamprajñata samadhi.

Samprajñata Samadhi

"Samprajñata samadhi is that which is accompanied by reasoning [vitarka], reflection [vichara], bliss [ananda] and sense of pure being [asmita]". Although it leads to chittanirodhavritti, the inhibition of the waves in the chitta, samprajñata samadhi is not that state–at least not fully. For it even to occur a great deal of the mind-waves must have gone into abeyance; still, it is not asamprajñata samadhi which is the full inhibition of all vrittis. It is, however, a genuine state of samadhi and a prerequisite for asamprajñata samadhi. For this reason we should analyse its characteristics. Although, as previously mentioned, many of the vrittis are inhibited, in samprajñata samadhi the vrittis of vitarka, vichara, ananda, and asmita may occur or be found underlying the consciousness of the yogi. We will consider each in turn.

Vitarka literally means reasoning or discussion–even argument. Within samprajñata samadhi it means the capacity for rational concepts to arise in a reflective or illuminating stream. I say "concepts" because words in the sense of internal silent speaking do not occur in samprajñata samadhi. Ordinary thinking is suppressed (actually superseded) in samprajñata samadhi, and the yogi's intelligence functions much further down the "thought chain" in simple, direct concepts.

That is, in samprajñata samadhi there is non-verbal reasoning, but not thinking in the ordinary meaning of silent internal verbalisation or "talking to oneself." This is important to know, because if inner verbalisation occurs it is a sign that our diving consciousness has begun to float up towards ordinary consciousness and that meditation needs to be induced again. What does all this mean practically? It means, for example, that if the light goes on in the room we will conceptualise that it has come on, further conceptualise that it cannot go on of its own accord, and conceptualise that someone may have entered the room. Then we will open our eyes to see who is there. Or, if we are meditating and the whole room begins to shake, the concepts of earthquake and the need to go to a safer place will arise. But in both instances only the concepts–not words–will arise if samprajñata samadhi is still being retained.

The practical value of this is that what we might call root-reason continues in samprajñata samadhi. And this can be to our benefit, obviously. When the doorbell or the telephone rings we are aware of it and also aware as to whether we need bother to answer or not. A momentary "discussion" in the form of a chain of conceptualisations may occur, but still the primary meditation-samadhi state is retained. This then leads us to realise that in time, with practice and progress, the state of samprajñata samadhi may be maintained even outside meditation–virtually all the time. This possibility was referred to by Ramana Maharshi: "Better than spells of meditation is one continuous current, steady as a stream, or downward flow of oil" (Verse seven ofUpadesha Saram–The Essence of Instruction). Meditation opens the door to this possibility.

Vichara means deliberation or reflection. Whereas vitarka is the power of conceptualisation related to outer phenomena, vichara relates to inner happenings during meditation such as inner distractions, the involuntary out-turning of the mind, or movement of the mind in a wrong direction such as outlined by Ramana Maharshi in section 2:16 of Spiritual Instruction: "It is important for one who is established in his Self (atma nishta) to see that he does not swerve in the least from this absorption. By swerving from his true nature he may see before him bright effulgences, etc., or hear (unusual) sounds or regard as real the visions of gods appearing within or outside himself. He should not be deceived by these and forget himself." When any of these things occur in samprajñata samadhi, the concept-reflection or non-verbal comprehension of their nature arises and we consciously stop, turn away, or reverse them. For example, when a memory of something arises we realise that it is a distraction and refuse to ruminate over it; when we find our mind floating up and out of meditation we consciously induce meditation again. And if experiences of the kind mentioned by Ramana Maharshi occur we ignore them or stop them. Vichara is not only conceptualisation of a subtle sort, it is also a subtle form of will which can manifest as a deliberate in-turning of the mind for the continuance of meditation. Vichara also develops our capacity for objectivity of mind, even outside meditation. This greatly contributes to our inner peace and the ability to intelligently respond to the situations of daily outer life.

Ananda is internal bliss, or joy. Meditation produces profound peace and relief from the internal effects or ravages of the outer storms of life. When this great peace and ease of heart are experienced in meditation, the experience of bliss–the "hem of the garment" of the Self–is not far away. Although there is indeed a state beyond bliss as an experience–asamprajñata samadhi–still ananda is a legitimate component of samprajñata samadhi.

Asmita is I-am-ness, the sense of individuality, of pure being, the feeling of "I exist." In meditation the yogi comes to be absorbed in this awareness of simple being, of I-am-ness. Yogic texts utilise the term asmita samadhi to denote what Sivananda says is the "superconscious state immediately below asamprajñata [samadhi] with the only or sole feeling of aham asmi: 'I am' or 'I exist.'" Vyasa comments: "Having discovered the self which is subtle as an atom, he should be conscious of 'I-am' alone." "This is meditation on its most refined cause, with everything else gone," adds Shankara. That is, there is no thought involving a defining or descriptive-adjectival condition, such as "I am sitting," "I am young," "I am serious," or "I amenlightened." Nothing whatsoever of the yogi's makeup or experience impinges on the pure "I am" awareness–not even "I amaware." Just the pure consciousness of consciousness itself in the form of the true self, or spirit, prevails in samprajñata samadhi. This is made possible by meditation.

Vitarka, vichara, ananda, and asmita may also be looked upon as the steps of samprajñata samadhi leading to asamprajñata samadhi. They are legitimate stages of deep yogic experience, both vital and valid and not to be scorned. So it is important that the yogi not become impatient and try to "go beyond them," for they alone are what leads us beyond. "There is no reason why the samadhi should not be in the form of 'I-am,' because this is meditation on its most refined cause, with everything else gone" (Shankara). "Of these, the first samadhi–with vitarka–is associated with all four. The second–with vichara–is without the verbal associations of the first. The third–with ananda–is without the subtle associations of the second. The fourth, being pure 'I-am,' is without the association of ananda. All these samadhis rest on an object" (Vyasa). That is: "In this sequence of four [stages], an earlier one is associated with the qualities of all the later ones, and a later one is without the qualities of any earlier one....Lest from the expression 'I am' it might be supposed that among these samadhis there is one without an object, he says, 'All these rest on an object.' It might be thought that 'I-am' is something without any idea in it. But it is not so,.... And so he will say later, '"I-am" is a feeling [bhava]'" (Shankara).

Lest we think that samprajñata samadhi and its most refined state of pure "I am"-ness is utter blankness or experience of nothing, Vyasa states that all the four stages of samprajñata samadhi, including the final one, "rest on an object."

This highest (or deepest) stage of samprajñata samadhi is not the experience of void, but of one's own true self in the form of consciousness. The stages of vitarka, vichara, and ananda "rest" upon the most subtle components of our relative existence, the causal levels that are so rarefied that they are naturally mistaken for the consciousness of the self. But when they are transcended, the "sense of pure being"–asmita–alone remains as the spirit rests (is centered) within its own self/nature, experiencing itself alone. So Vyasa later comments that "asmita is a sense," the most subtle sense or awareness of pure being.

Stating the practical value or effect of samprajñata samadhi, Vyasa says: "The samadhi in the one-pointed mind makes clear the object as it is, destroys the taints, loosens the karma-bonds, and brings the state of inhibition [chittavrittinirodhah] into view; it is called samprajñata [cognitive]." Shankara comments that Vyasa is speaking of a "one-pointedness where there is no subjection to a state."

Since we are so egoically obsessed with the need to be or have the "highest" and the "best," we are in danger of putting little value on our experience of samprajñata samadhi during our practice of meditation and trying to force or push ourselves "higher" or "deeper" into asamprajñata samadhi. Not only is such an attempt futile, we are indulging in foolish disregard of something that is supremely valuable and worthy of all respect. Vyasa warns us from this error by assuring us that "the omission of the word 'all' [in speaking of the suppression of vrittis in the Yoga Sutra 1:2] shows that samprajñata samadhi also is yoga." Shankara, commenting on this statement, says that yoga "is well known to include meditation on objects."

Although the highest yoga (asamprajñata samadhi) is without objects, the lesser yoga (samprajñata samadhi) does include awareness of the subtle inner functions already listed. Therefore he continues, commenting on Vyasa: "He has not said that cognitive samadhi is putting down the mental process entirely....Cognitive samadhi is still accompanied by certain mental objects." The stages of meditation leading to transcendence (asamprajñata samadhi) are also yoga. Furthermore, they are of great practical value.

Vyasa assures us in the previously-cited comment that meditation in the form of samprajñata samadhi:

- Makes clear the object as it is;
- Destroys the taints [kleshas];
- Loosens the karma-bonds;
- Brings the state of inhibition [chittavrittinirodhah] into view.

As we say in our American slang, this is nothing to be sneezed at! These four effects of samprajñata samadhi are directly linked to its four stages or qualities: vitarka, vichara, ananda, and asmita. Moreover, these effects are not confined to the time of meditation practice, but extend into the daily life of the yogi as well. So the practicer of meditation must greatly value even the "lesser" stages of meditation which produce these marvelous results so effortlessly.

The vitarka–subtle reasoning power–which is produced and developed by meditation practice "makes clear the object as it is." That is, it enables the yogi, both in and out of meditation, to see clearly whatever comes into the purview of his mind-consciousness. He sees the truth of a thing–both its subtle behind-the-scenes nature and purpose as well as its ultimate truth as a manifestation of Pure Consciousness: God.

The vichara (reflection) capacity which is produced and developed by meditation practice "destroys the taints" known askleshas in the Yoga Sutras 2:2,3: "The samadhi produced by meditation is for the removal of the kleshas. The kleshas are: ignorance, egoism, attraction and repulsion for objects, and fear of death." These kleshas are the root causes of all the afflictions and misery encountered in human life. And meditation dissolves them all.

The ananda-bliss-which is produced and developed by meditation practice "loosens the karma-bonds." This is because desire for happiness or joy is the root motivation of all actions producing karma. But when that ananda is gained through the practice of meditation, the compulsion towards material, external actions for egoic attainment ceases, for fulfillment is found. The asmita--awareness of pure being-which is produced and developed by meditation practice "brings the state of inhibition [chittavrittinirodhah] into view." That is, it gives a touch of the ultimate state of asamprajñata samadhi ("brings it into view") and impels the consciousness onward to that higher state. All these effects come from a great deal of meditation-not just after a few days' practice. But the results are assured to the faithful yogi.

Asamprajñata Samadhi

"Asampajñata samadhi was defined in the words, 'Yoga is the cessation (nirodha) of modifications (vritti) in the mind-substance (chitta),'" says Shankara. And Vyasa: "Asamprajñata samadhi is when there is inhibition of all mental processes." Asamprajñata samadhi is yoga in the most absolute sense. It is both the end of yoga and yoga itself. This of course must become our permanent state. Therefore practice is still needed even after its attainment.

In contrasting the two types of samadhi, samprajñata and asamprajñata, Shankara avers: "The definition as inhibition [of vrittis] applies exactly to asamprajñata samadhi, but only loosely to samprajñata samadhi" since in samprajñata samadhi, though there is a great–almost total–inhibition of the vrittis, still some do occur as contrasted with asamprajñata samadhi in which absolutely no vrittis arise. And further: "Asamprajñata samadhi cannot be defined by anything else except inhibition. Inhibition alone is its definition because nothing else is there, whereas samprajñata samadhi is definable in terms of special characteristics like verbal [*i.e.*, conceptual] associations....It is settled that asamprajñata samadhi is defined by the bare word 'inhibition.'...The commentator will sum up later in these words: 'It is asamprajñata in the sense that in it no thing is cognised [samprajñayate]: this yoga is inhibition of the mental process.'" He also has written in his Yoga Sutra commentary: "The one-pointed [ekagra] state of the mind is a stream of similar thoughts....The inhibited [niruddha] state is a mind empty of thoughts." And: "In inhibition [nirodh] the mind is not restricted to a particular object, for there is no subject for an object."

In Yoga Sutra 1:18 Patanjali speaks of asamprajñata samadhi in a most interesting manner: "The other is when by practice [of samprajñata samadhi] the last vestiges of the contents [the vrittis] of the mind cease [or are dropped]." "The other" is asamprajñata samadhi, but it is significant that he neither names it nor speaks of it as being produced or even occurring by the cessation of all vrittis in the chitta. This is because it is not an entity, thing, or even–speaking precisely–a state, but a result of the cessation of all such things and their experience and effect. Vyasa puts it this way: "In this state [of asamprajñata samadhi] what remains is samskaras, and it is the seedless [nirbija] samadhi.

There is no cognition of anything in it, so it is asamprajñata. This yoga is inhibition of the mental processes." Shankara, commenting on this says: "The meaning is, that here the seed is gone; in this all the seeds of taint and so on are gone."

Also, by using the expression "the other" for asamprajñata samadhi Patanjali is following the lead of the Advaita Vedanta philosophy in which Reality is not designated as One, but rather only as Not Two [Advaita]. This is because asamprajñata samadhi is the eternal, ineradicable state of the spirit-of consciousness itself. Having always been, it can neither be attained nor produced. It always IS, for it is the state of I AM.

Samprajñata samadhi is savikalpa samadhi, and asamprajñata samadhi is nirvikalpa samadhi. Savikalpa means "with content" and nirvikalpa means "without content." By "content" is meant impressions in the mind that will manifest subsequently in the form of positive states of consciousness and positive karmas, and the experiences of objects, however subtle. Savikalpa samadhi produces something, whereas nirvikalpa samadhi is the cessation and prevention of all "somethings."

The following valuable simple exposition of the various yogic states is given by A. W. Chadwick in A Sadhu's Reminiscences of Ramana Maharshi: "Savikalpa Samadhi is the state of deep meditation when one is sunk in peace but still retains the consciousness of one's identity.

One knows that one is meditating and can still consciously continue one's Sadhana. InNirvikalpa Samadhi one has attained to a state where the identity has been lost and sunk entirely in the highest Self. However long it may last it is only temporary, one must return eventually to one's normal state of consciousness.

One is unable to function in this state and so long as it lasts one is in a state of trance. It is usually preliminary to the final state [of Sahaja Samadhi]. Sahaja Samadhi is the final and most blessed state, the goal of all Yogis. In this state the individual has become completely merged in the Supreme Self. His identity which became lost in Nirvikalpa Samadhi has become enlarged and is now the Supreme Self and knows itself as such. Trances are no longer necessary, a person can still carry on with the ordinary day to day business but he no longer identifies himself with the activities, but watches them like a dreamer watching a dream. There is no more to do, and no more to be attained. This is the Supreme State of Absolute Bliss."

In samprajñata samadhi we experience the self only, and in asamprajñata samadhi we experience God, the Self of our self. Saint Paul speaks of it in this way: "For now we see [in samprajñata samadhi as though] through a glass, darkly; but then [in asamprajñata samadhi] face to face: now [in samprajñata samadhi] I know in part; but then [in asamprajñata samadhi] shall I know even as also I am known". In the matter of asamprajñata samadhi we are not talking about an attainment, but a rediscovery, a remembering–literally a realisation. Not being the result of an action it is therefore permanent and ineradicable.

CHAPTER

6

Clinical Hypnosis and Patanjali Yoga Sutras

CONSCIOUSNESS AND ALTERED STATES OF CONSCIOUSNESS

Consciousness can be defined as the subjective awareness of the momentary experience interpreted in the context of personal memory and present state. Altered state of consciousness is also defined in terms of a change in the subjective experience. One popular definition is the one given by Tart in 1990. He defines the altered state of consciousness as one in which the individual feels a qualitative shift in his pattern of mental functioning; there is a change in the qualities of mental processes. It is not just defined as a quantitative shift, in terms of more or less alert, more or less visual imagery, etc.

This definition highlights that primary phenomenal consciousness; which is awareness of a changed pattern of subjective experience; and reflective consciousness, in which a cognitive judgement must be passed so as to recognise that the experience is different from normal; are both involved in the altered state of consciousness.

Altered states of consciousness or trance state have also been understood as a deviation from the normal states of consciousness. It has been understood as a state in which the world or the self tend to be misrepresented. This is caused by an internal or external change in the organism's biological makeup and it alters the representational relations and hence is not a functional, original or permanent state of the organisms' consciousness. An altered state of consciousness is thus, due to a change in the representational state of consciousness and is not restricted to any specific cognitive, affective of sensory modality, but is a combination of them, and it is a temporary phenomenon.

According to this understanding of altered states of consciousness or trance state, hypnosis can be considered as one, because it changes the background mechanisms of consciousness, as strong and multiple changes in conscious experiences are experienced as hypnotic suggestions.

Hypnosis through the Ages

Hypnosis is derived from the Greek root hypnos, which means to sleep. Even the origins of the word means to sleep, hypnosis is not a state of sleeping. The trance in hypnosis resembles sleep, but this trance is different from the other states of consciousness (awake, sleep, and dream states).

Although it is Anton Mesmer, who is credited for the origin of hypnosis, it is not true. Two-thousand years before Mesmer, techniques of induction were being used by ancient Egyptian and Greek priests. There is evidence of Egyptian priests performing death and rebirth rituals in what they called as "Temples of Sleep." Drugs and psychedelics were used to assist the process. Those who lived through the experience were said to "have experienced other levels of reality while being out of the physical body." Hypnosis is as old as time and has been employed in all parts of the world in some form or the other.

James Braid used the term hypnosis derived from the word hypnos, as he thought that hypnosis was similar to sleep. He developed the eye fixation technique of inducing relaxation and called it hypnosis. Abbe Faria, a Catholic priest, was a pioneer in the scientific study of hypnosis. It was him who stated that it was not animal magnetism that was involved in the cure, but suggestion. Later, Braid recognised that hypnosis is similar to meditation in both, the psychological and physiological aspects.

He defined hypnotism as a state of focussed attention upon a single idea or mental image. In his view, since hypnosis was the state of focused attention, it was fundamentally the opposite of normal sleep. After he recognised his error (of believing that hypnosis was similar to sleep), he tried to change the name to monoedisimo, which means a concentration on one side. The term hypnosis, even though a misnomer, still persists.

In 1854, James Esdaile, a Scottish surgeon, was working in India with the East India Company. While here, he performed hundreds of minor and major surgical procedures on Indians under Mesmeric anesthesia. His book describes hundreds of operations that he performed under this technique, including amputations of the legs, removal of tumors, and other comparable surgeries. He even noted the dwindling of surgical shock in his patients. In his book, Hypnosis in Medicine and Surgery, 1957, he describes that he or his assistants would induce hypnosis (mesmerised) the patients in the morning, and would leave them in a cataleptic state. He would then return later and operate. When Esdaile returned to England and shared his experiences, he was, unfortunately ridiculed and ostracised by his colleagues.

The first scientific text on hypnosis, Suggestive Therapeutics was published in 1886 by Bernheim. Bernheim observed the work of Dr. Ambroise-Auguste Liebault, a French physician. Liebault became interested in hypnosis after reading Braid's work, but in order to avoid being discredited, he worked pro bono. Bernhiem and Liebault then began to work together, treating patients.

Ernst Simmel, a German psychoanalyst began using hypnosis for the treatment of war neurosis or shell shock. He called his technique hypnoanalysis. In hypnoanalysis, hypnosis was combined with the psychodynamic techniques.

During World War II Grinker and Spiegel used barbiturates to induce a state of drug hypnosis in order to bring traumatic material to the surface. Hypnosis has since been playing an important part in the treatment of combat fatigue and other neuroses. The most important development to come out of the world wars was the merger of hypnotic techniques with psychoanalysis. This development revived a great deal of interest in hypnosis and led to the publication of various books with hypnosis and suggestibility as the subject matter.

Hypnosis has since been recognised as a treatment method by the American Medical Association (in 1958). There are now several journals devoted exclusively to the experimental and clinical applications of hypnosis. These include, but are not limited to The American Journal of Clinical Hypnosis, The British Journal of Medical Hypnotism, The Journal of Clinical and Experimental Hypnosis.

Theories of Hypnosis

The phenomena associated with hypnosis are explained through two main types of theories. These are referred to as state and non-state theories. A key debate in hypnosis had been between the state and non-state theorists. According to the state theorists, hypnotic inductions produce an altered state of consciousness, which is associated with an altered state of brain function. The response to suggestion is also due to special processes such as dissociation or other altered states of consciousness. The non-state theorists however, are of the view that participants respond to suggestion without hypnosis and that suggestibility can be modified by drugs and psychological procedures; and the participants in hypnosis are actively engaged to be in a trance state. They also hold the belief that responses to suggestions are a product of normal psychological processes such as attitudes, expectancies, and motivations.

Hilgard's neo-dissociation theory of hypnosis is a classic state theory. It proposes that hypnotic phenomena are produced through dissociation within high level control systems. This means that the hypnotic suggestion is said to split the functioning of the executive control system into different streams. Part of the executive control system functions normally, but is unable to represent itself in conscious awareness due to the presence of an amnesic barrier. The hypnotic suggestions act on the dissociated part of the executive control system and the subject is aware of the result of the suggestion and not the process by which they came about.

Neuro-physiological theories of hypnosis propose that high hypnotisable people have better executive function than low hypnotisable people. Since they have better executive functioning, they are able to deploy their attention in different ways. One model of hypnosis characterises it as a change in bran function. This neurophysiological account emphasizes that the changes in the way the attentional control system operates in hypnosis makes the subject more suggestible.

Social cognitive theory of hypnosis argues that the experience of effortlessness in hypnosis results from participant's motivated tendencies to interpret hypnotic suggestions as not requiring active planning and effort (*i.e.* the experience of effortlessness stems from an attributional error).

The attribution of volition depends on the kind of response-set which has been put into place, and if a hypnotic response-set is in place then volition is attributed externally. This means that the effortlessness in hypnosis comes about when individuals expect things to be effortless, and "decide" (more or less consciously) to respond along with suggestions.

One important factor to note when considering socio-cognitive hypnosis theories of this sort is that they do not imply that subjects are always "faking," or not really experiencing an involuntary hypnotic response. Although these models use terms such as "role enactment" or "self-presentation" they are still entirely consistent with the notion that hypnotised participants have unusual experiences.

The ecological theory of hypnosis is based on Shor's idea that the depth of hypnotic trance is related to the degree to which the participant loses awareness of the distinction between imagination and reality. This distinction is termed as the generalised reality orientation.

Ego-psychological theory distinguishes between primary processes (emotional, holistic, illogical, unconscious, developmentally immature) and secondary processes (affect-free, analytical, logical, conscious, developmentally mature). Whereas normal adult functioning is biased towards secondary processing the induction of hypnosis makes the subject "let go" of some secondary process activity. Critically, this theory is not as well-specified as some other cognitive theories, and is thus not as easily testable or falsifiable.

The third way research in hypnosis understands the phenomena in hypnosis as both a state of cognitive change that involves basic mechanisms of cognition and consciousness, and as a product of social interaction as the hypnotist and the subject come together for a specific purpose within a wider socio-cultural context. The third way theories include the integrative cognitive theory which makes a distinction between being in a mental state and being aware of being in that state. An emphasis is placed on perception and consciousness. It includes the dissociated control theory concept which suggests that responses are facilitated by an inhibition of high-level attention and the response set idea that suggested that involuntariness is an attribution about the causes of behaviour.

The Trance in Hypnosis

It is difficult to define a hypnotic trance state, but it can be inferred from hypersuggestibility, passivity, disinclination to talk, and fixed facial expressions, feelings of relaxation, unreality, automaticity and compulsion, alterations in body image, and unusual sensations have been reported to accompany hypnotic trance. The hypnotic state has been described as one in which there is focused attention, concentration in which learning is maximized, alterations in self-awareness, a state of internally focused absorption and the suspension of normal reality testing, alterations in perceptions.

The trance in hypnosis is characterised by a quiet, calm and peaceful mind. There exists a general sense of wellbeing. They describe it as a state of alert restfulness as the person is awake but the state is more like sleep than awake. The subjective time moves slowly, and the distinction between the present, past, and future is lost. There is a shift of space location and one can experience oneself at several different locations in space. The depth of trance may be mild, moderate, or intense in depth.

Initially, the pulse rate and blood pressure rise, but they soon go below the resting levels. The respiratory rate also first rises and then falls below the resting level. The metabolic rate falls steeply and it may fall below the level of sleep. The body and face seem flushed as the peripheral flow of blood increases. There is also a decline in the plasma coritsol levels and there is increased functioning in both the hemispheres of the brain.

Lethargy is present in a light hypnosis state. It is characteristic in this state that muscles contract at the slightest touch, friction, pressure, or massage. This contraction can be restricted, by the by, the repetition of the stimuli that caused it. In this state of light trance, the subject appears to be in deep sleep, the eyes are closed or half closed and the face is expressionless. The body appears to be in a state of complete collapse with the head thrown back, and the arms and legs hang loose, dropping heavily down.

Catalepsy characterises a deeper level of trance and in this the subject becomes rigidly fixed in the position in which they were in while they were entering catalepsy. Whether it is standing, or sitting, or kneeling. Arms or legs can be raised and will remain in that position.

Since a trance state is also described as one in which there is a "heightened focus of attention or concentration on internal or external cues" one can say that hypnosis is an altered state of consciousness or a trance state.

In this trance state, perception is clarified. What an individual perceives is colored by various projections of the mind. They refuse to accept perceptual clarity and the perception of reality is through these projections, in the hypnotic trance state however, reality is perceived free of the projections.

Consciousness In Yoga

Consciousness in yoga can be conceptualised as William James' idea of consciousness. William James compared consciousness to a stream that was unbroken and continuous. This stream however, goes through constant changes and shifts and Patanjali yoga sutra states that there are seven states of consciousness orSaptadha prantabhumihi pragyana.

These seven states are as follows:

1. Awake
2. Sleep
3. Dream
4. Turya
5. The fifth state is defined as "abiding in mere non-duality, with all distinction and division extinguished, he is seen as one asleep"
6. The sixth state is described as where he dwells "without knot," liberated while living and without conception or ideation
7. The seventh state is the state of enlightenment, which is the state of liberation without the body.

The turya state has been described as a tranquil settlement in the state of liberation and the state of witness in action. The state of turya has been explained in the Mandukya Upanishad as:

"...that which has no parts, soundless, the incomprehensible, beyond all senses, the cessation of all phenomena, all blissful and non-dual AUM, is the Fourth, and verily it is the same as Atman. He who knows this, merges his self in the supreme self - the individual in the total."

Since there is a distorted sense of self in this state, which is a misrepresentation, this state can be considered as an altered state of consciousness.

The altered state of consciousness or trance state of yoga is that of Samadhi. It is described by the phrase sat-chit-ananda, which translates to truth-consciousness-bliss. This relates to a different realm of experience which is possible to describe only by metaphors and paradoxes.

According to Patanjali yoga sutras, Samadhi is the goal of yoga. It can be defined as the pointless point of consciousness beyond which nothing else remains. It is the deepest level of consciousness where even the sense of individuality does not remain. From the literature reviewed it can be seen that the trance states of yoga and hypnosis have certain similarities. Trance in both the states is associated with relaxation, disinclination to talk, unreality, misrepresentation, alterations in perception, increased concentration, suspension of normal reality testing, and the temporary nature of the phenomena. Yoga can be considered to be a form of hypnosis and many similarities between the trance state of hypnosis and yoga have been noted. While yogis are credited with performing difficult tasks like walking over burning coal, or being able to lie on nails, individuals under the hypnotic trance are reported to have "heavy weights on their abdomen while lying stretched in midair with supports only at his heads or ankles." Apart from this, not much research has been carried out, which investigates the similarities if any in the trance of yoga and hypnosis. In this study, I aim to aim to fill this gap literature by comparing the trance state in hypnosis and yoga. Along with this I will also focus on the therapeutic techniques of yoga and hypnosis.

Research Design

In this study, whose aim is to investigate the similarities between hypnosis and yoga in terms of the altered states of consciousness, regression and therapeutic value, a qualitative design is used.

A qualitative study is one that provides an in-depth understanding and interpretation of phenomena by learning about the social and material circumstances, and histories. A qualitative design is suited for this study as it helps to investigate whether or not there are similarities between the trance states of yoga and that of hypnosis. The qualitative methodology also helps to explore the historical, philosophical, and scientific roots of yoga and hypnosis and the conceptualisation of the trance states in them. The study uses a pragmatic approach as methods and procedures that work best for answering the research question have been employed.

Research Questions

Broad Research Question: To investigate the similarities between yoga and hypnosis.

Specific Research Question: To investigate the similarities between Patanjali yoga sutras and hypnosis in terms of the altered states of consciousness, and their therapeutic value.

Sample

The sample consists of a text on Patanjali yoga sutra: Four Chapters on Freedom: A Commentary on the Yoga Sutras of Patanjali, by Swami Satyananda. The book is published by the Bihar School of Yoga, which is the world's first yoga university. The Bihar School of Yoga was founded by Swami Satyananda Saraswati in the year 1964. The book, Four Chapters on Freedom is a text used for the courses in the university, and is a widely accepted text on Patanjali yoga sutras. This is the reason this text is selected for analysis.

Data collection

The following serve as data for the study:

- The text on Patanjali yoga sutra.
- Discussion of findings with expert: Findings obtained from the thematic analysis are communicated to an expert and discussed with her. This discussion provides insights, which are incorporated into the study.

Data Analysis

Thematic analysis is the method of analysis for the first phase of the study. Thematic analysis is defined as a general method of analysis of text. It is a method for "identifying, analysing and reporting patterns within data." There are six steps in the through which thematic analysis progresses. In the first phase the familiarisation with the data is achieved, followed by generation of initial codes, following, which there is the search for themes, which are then reviewed, defined and named and then the report is written.

Following the same process, in the first phase Four Chapters on Freedom: A Commentary on the Yoga Sutras of Patanjali, is read to become familiar with the text. This is followed by an initial coding which leads to the formation of themes. The themes are then reviewed and then defined and named. Through this process meaning units are created, which describe and explain each of the phenomena under study. These are then used to form themes, which illustrate each of the phenomena.

In the second phase of the study, the themes generated through the thematic analysis of the text are compared with the concepts in hypnosis to investigate whether or not there are similarities between the phenomena in Patanjali yoga sutras and phenomena in hypnosis.

Issues of trustworthiness and process of validation:

- The themes obtained from the analysis were finalised after discussion with a student pursuing her Masters

in Psychological Research Methodology who went through relevant passages from the text independently
- The findings were discussed with the supervisor and an expert in the field of yoga which provided further insight. This served as a method of triangulation
- Peer debriefing: A competent peer was given regular progress reports of the research
- A paper trail of the documents used for analysis, and the different stages of analysis is maintained and is available on request.

Analysis Of Results And Discussion

The text which was analysed, Four Chapters on Freedom: Commentary on the Yoga Sutras of Patanjali by Swami Satyananda Sarswati was published in 1976.

This book is a commentary on the yoga sutras written by the sage Patanjali. Sutra means thread and it is implied, by the use of this word, that the written verses carry and underlying, continuous and unbroken thought. The various ideas in the sutras connect with each other and one thought leads to the next resulting in a complete philosophy.

The yoga sutras of Patanjali consist of 196 sutras, which are organised into four chapters.

These are:

- *Samadhi Pada:* This consists of 51 verses and is the chapter on Samadhi.
- *Sadhana Pada:* This consists of 55 verses and is the chapter on practice.
- *Vibhooti Pada:* This chapter discusses various psychic powers and consists of 56 verses.
- *Kaivalya Pada:* It the chapter on isolation or aloneness. It consists of 34 verses.

From the thematic analysis, it was found that there are similarities between the trance state in hypnosis and yoga.

These similarities are found in terms of:

- The induction and deepening of the trance states in hypnosis and that of Samadhi
- The phenomena present in hypnosis and the siddhis obtained through Samadhi
- The therapeutic techniques and the therapeutic process in Patanjali's yoga sutra and hypnosis.

Along with the similarities between the two, there were many ideas in Patanjali yoga sutras which were found to be similar to psychological concepts.

Psychological Concepts in Patanjali Yoga Sutras

There are many ideas in Patanjali yoga sutras that are parallel to and resemble concepts that are present in psychology. The mind or chitta as described in Patanjali yoga sutras is said to be comprised of the conscious, subconscious and the unconscious. Patanjali yoga sutras also believe that self-realisation can take place only when the chitta vrittis cease their activity or when the chitta is no longer affected by the three gunas.

Only when there is a cessation of identification with the outside objective world, the mind is able to see things as they are. This is similar to the idea in psychology of the presence of schemas through which we make sense of the world. Schemas can be conceptualised as organised patterns of thought and behaviours or structures that organise our knowledge and assumptions about something that is used for interpreting and processing information.

They influence our attention to a situation and also influence what we look for in situations. It is the schemas that guide our thinking and information processing. All the information that is received from the external world is interpreted through the schemas we hold. In order to gain an objective understanding, one must look at this information outside of the schemas. This is essentially the same idea that is present in Patanjali yoga sutras as well. The mind, Patanjali explains, is colored and conditioned by its likes, dislikes, and false beliefs. It further explains that the external reality is superimposed with the modifications of the mind. This can result in misidentification leading to feelings of joy, sadness, fear, like, dislike, etc., Suffering is a result of the identification of the modification of the mind with the external object. In order to overcome suffering this association has to be broken.

Patanjali yoga sutras also hold that memory is made up of past impressions. Smriti, it describes as an independent awareness on which impressions are embedded. It also believes that even if the past clears up, the smriti remains. Thus we see that smriti is analogous to schemas as schemas too, are mental structures that help us organise information regarding the external world. They are cognitive representations of the self which guide the kind of attention paid to external events and the meaning that they convey.

The modifications of the mind, according to the yoga sutras are of five kinds (depending on the sense that is responsible for the perception) and are either painful or pleasurable (there is a liking of the pleasurable and a disliking of the painful). This holds that an object or event in itself is not painful or pleasurable, but it is the mind that makes it so.

It is the attachment that one has towards objects that causes attraction and repulsion towards them. Abandonment of this attachment or the process of detachment gives rise to freedom from this attraction or repulsion, thereby helping in controlling the pleasure and pain one experiences. This is the same as the concept of cognitive theory and cognitive hypnotherapy. Cognitive theory posits that people tend to perceive and interpret situations in characteristic ways that colour their feelings and shape their behaviours. People often have spontaneous, automatic thoughts about their past, current or future situations. People are not conscious of the automatic thoughts but of the emotions arising from them.

These arise from the beliefs and ideas that are embedded in the mental structures of the mind. These are called schemas. These schemas have the ability to bias processing of information and external events are colored by the schemas which guide the individual. This makes the individual infer an external event as positive or negative, pleasurable, or painful.

The yoga sutras also explain the yogic theory of perception. This holds that even though the object is one, it is perceived differently at different times and by different people depending on the difference in mental conditions. It is this difference in perception that makes object capable of inducing pleasure and pain and suffering. Once the perception is cleansed of one's mental modifications external events fail to evoke pain and suffering in the in the individual. This is similar to the principle of cognitive behaviour therapy.

The yoga sutras also hold the concept of conscious and subconscious memory. Conscious memory involves the recollection of things already experienced. This is different from subconscious memory that refers to the memory that one does not consciously remember. This may present itself in dreams and the memories that are revealed there are memories of actual events that are not distorted.

The sutras thus, are of the opinion that conscious memories are distorted due to our impressions are remembered as such and not as what the reality was. This is in line with the idea of memory being a reconstructive process.

The yoga sutras also discuss pain and its cause. They explain that pain is not in the present but is rooted in the past. Klesha is the agony that is present in our very being. According to them, everyone feels pain but everyone is not aware of it.

Pain is thought to be at the bottom of everything and Patanjali also talks of three different types of pain:

- The first pain is change, life changes to death
- The second is acute anxiety, achievement, success and love give rise to anxiety at some time or the other;

- The third pain is habit, we become used to things and are then afraid of losing them.

Hypnosis and Patanjali Yoga Sutras

The process of attaining the trance state in hypnosis is referred to as the induction process. One of them is the eye fixation method. In the eye, fixation method is a type of hypnotic induction method that people associate most with hypnosis. In this method, the client is instructed to maintain a fixed gaze on an object. This could be any object, a spot on the wall, the hand of the hypnotist, a finger held in front of the client's eyes, or even, the flame of a lamp. This method is similar to the technique described in the yoga sutras, wherein the aspirant concentrates on an object, internal or external, which could be the image of a deity, a flame, the tip of the nose or even concentrating between the eyebrows to attain Samadhi.

Similarities in the Phenomena

In the trance of hypnosis, there is a shift in the perception of the external world and the internal environment. Some of these changes can be compared to the siddhis described in the Patanjali yoga sutras. Subjective time appears to move slowly and an hour may appear to have been only a few minutes. Memories of remote events of the past are recalled with uncanny accuracy. During hypnosis, the power of selected groups of muscles can be increased, which is the same as the attainment of strength. This increase in strength can be maintained after the trance state through the use of post-hypnotic suggestion. The body temperature can be made to increase in the trance of hypnosis; this is found in the yoga sutras as well. The action of the organs can be changed, and this is a siddhi too. Hearing is said, can be made more acute in the trance of hypnosis, this is analogous to the siddhi of divine hearing. Thus we see that there are indeed similarities in the phenomena of hypnosis with the siddhis described in the Patanjali yoga sutras.

Therapeutic Process and Techniques

Hypnosis and hypnotherapy is a paradigmatic phenomenon. It challenges fundamental assumptions of self and reality. An individual's perceptions and beliefs can be overturned through hypnosis and hypnotherapy.

Hypnotherapy also believes that schemas or cognitive structures regulate psychological functioning or adaptation and give meaning to contextual relationships. Assignment of meaning at the conscious and unconscious level activates behavioural, emotional, and other strategies of adaptation. One of the essential axioms of hypnotherapy is that meanings do not always represent reality but are a construction of a given context or goal and are subject to cognitive distortions. Some individuals are vulnerable to cognitive distortions. This is the same as the mental modifications that influence the perception of reality as explained by the yoga sutras; and the techniques of Patanjali yoga sutra and hypnosis allow access to processes below the threshold of awareness, which helps in the restricting of non-conscious cognitions.

Like the techniques described in the yoga sutras for therapeutic benefits, hypnosis too induces relaxation, which is effective in reducing anxiety. It also promotes ego strengthening through the repetition of positive suggestions to oneself that get embedded in the unconscious mind. These then exert an automatic influence on feelings, thoughts, and behaviours. This enhances one's self-confidence and self-worth.

Hypnosis and the techniques of yoga sutras facilitate divergent thinking, it maximizes awareness among several levels of brain functioning. They both have a direct impact on focus of attention and concentration. They also help in directing attention to wider experiences such as feelings of warmth, feeling happy, feeling of contentment, and general feeling of wellbeing. They serve to expand these experiences in the present, past, and future. These facilitate in the reconstruction of dysfunctional realities.

Even though modern psychotherapy adopts a curative paradigm and the yoga surtras of Patanjali operates through a preventive paradigm, there are similarities in the therapeutic techniques, and the therapeutic gain obtained from hypnosis and Patanjali yoga sutras. Since it has already been pointed out that ancient Indian paradigm of consciousness is holistic and is related to mental health, the trance in yoga can be used in modern psychotherapeutic processes.

The indeed hypnotic similarities in yoga with regard to the conceptualisation of consciousness and altered state of consciousness, the phenomena in the altered states of consciousness and the therapeutic benefits and the therapy process.

In India, the therapeutic process is closely linked to faith and hence it make sense to make use of the traditional therapeutic modalities in modern therapeutic paradigm.

CHAPTER

7

Patanjali's Conception of the Mind in Yoga

What is yoga? Despite the current popularity of yoga practice, few people, when pressed, seem capable of providing a satisfactory answer to this question. The complexity, subtlety and paradox inherent in the ancient tradition does not lend itself to an easy answer. At the beginning of the Yoga Sutra, however—in the second aphorism to be precise, Patanjali gives what seems to be a concise and definitive definition: "Yogas citta vritti nirodhah" That this is not the end of the matter—but rather the mere beginning of a long journey into esoteric realms of both theory and experience—becomes clear when one examines the bewildering variety of translations of this Sanskrit aphorism into English. "Yoga is a restriction of the fluctuations of consciousness... Yoga is the control of the thought waves in the mind....Yoga is restraining the activities of the mind.... Yoga is the process of ending the definitions of the field of consciousness... Yoga is the cessation of the misidentification with the modifications of the mind..."

Part of this difficulty lies in translation. As the "language of the gods", a sacred tongue consecrated to the transmission of spiritual truth, Sanskrit words do not easily find their equivalents in our modern secular English. Yet both the number of Sanskrit commentators over the centuries and the length of their works suggest that there is much more to it than that. Patanjali's aphorisms express in a succinct, elliptical style nuggets of truth gleaned from first hand experience.

Though taken as a whole the Yoga Sutra forms an integrated philosophy, its theoretical dimension depends upon direct encounter rather than speculative thought. The aphorisms emerge from a distillation of actual experience into language, a language eminently suited to contain the fruit of spiritual practice. Theory then builds upon language, attempting to formulate a complete metaphysics out of shimmering wisdom drawn from depths where no language could ever reach.

Not only does Patanjali's theoretical system result from experiential understanding, but it intends to ignite a similar fire for practice in the genuine seeker. To the aspirant who studies it carefully, it provides a map for accessing the spiritual reality directly. Its purpose is practical, not speculative or intellectual. The Yoga Sutra is a tool designed for use. An understanding of the metaphysics it teaches serves primarily to clarify the path towards the actual experience that gave birth to these structures in the first place. Theory is not enough. "Just as a good knowledge of culinary science does not satisfy hunger, neither will the benefits of yoga be realised fully by a mere understanding of the science of its practice." And so in this work Patanjali teaches a methodical yoga, a systematic approach oriented towards the pinnacle of spiritual practice: direct realisation of Ultimate Truth. This method begins and ends with the mind. For the mind is the primary tool the aspirant will employ. The mind is at the same time the seeker, the field of seeking and the ever elusive sought.

As Patanjali shows, the mind (or chitta) holds the key to Ultimate Reality. But the mind can serve either as doorway or barrier, a vehicle for spiritual liberation or an instrument of enslavement. So to return to the original question, "What is yoga?" and Patanjali's reply, "Yogas chittas vritti nirodhah", it is apparent what needs clarifying. Without an understanding of "chitta" or Patanjali's conception of the mind, we have little hope either of answering that question or grasping Patanjali's enigmatic statement. Patanjali's conception of the mind has profound philosophical and psychological implications. But most significantly, it places effective yoga practice in a clear framework, guiding the aspirant towards fruitful progress along the path of direct spiritual experience and ultimate liberation.

Before looking directly at Patanjali's model of the mind, it would be useful (though difficult) for us to put aside any assumptions we may be holding about the nature of the mind based on our cultural conditioning or educational background. It is good to approach Patanjali (and everything else) freshly. This is actually one of Patanjali's points. The residue of past experiences that the mind acquires through action in life functions like a distorted lens, preventing us from seeing anything as it truly is. What we want to see (or realise) more than anything else through our yoga practice is the nature of our True Identity. But too many things are clouding the picture. A kind of spiritual myopia blocks our awareness of our True Self. How this happens is precisely the issue Patanjali addresses in his conception of the mind.

If I discard all attachment to possessions, family, friends, occupation, preferences, aversions, education, culture, prejudices, belief systems... Who am I? What if I detach from my body too...? What am I then?

Patanjali provides a framework for understanding these questions. But it is important to remember that his conception of the mind, in all its detail of structure and function, is a model, not the thing itself. A model is like a map. And as this one derives from Patanjali's own experience, it is very useful to follow. However, as the well-known adage goes, "The map is not the territory." No matter how useful, it is good to hold this model (any model) lightly, not taking it so literally that its categories get reified into absolutes or dogma.

In Patanjali's system of duality, reality consists of two separate dimensions: purusha and prakriti. Purusha is pure consciousness, the transcendental Self, the immutable, eternal, attribute-less essence of life. Prakriti is creative energy—essentially everything else, not only physical matter in all its myriad manifestations but ideas, thoughts and subtle energy patterns.

All is Prakriti. The world as macrocosm and the mind as microcosm both belong to prakriti, though the essence of both is purusha. The mind—as everything else in the three worlds—has both purusha and prakriti aspects. Because purusha is without attributes, it is difficult to say much about it. It is absolutely beyond the grasp of our senses and intellect, not to mention language. Prakriti, however, can be described in precise detail, and is in the Yoga Sutra. As purusha is pure consciousness, so prakriti is absolute insentience.

All consciousness or awareness is the light of purusha shining through the forms of prakriti. Purusha is the witness: pure subject. Like the sun, the light of purusha shines upon the patterns of prakriti, making them luminous and apparent. As creative energy, prakriti is always moving, all manifestation never ceasing its dance of change and transformation. But despite this, the forms of prakriti in themselves remain devoid of consciousness. Prakriti is pure object, a shimmering mirror that the light of purusha illuminates with endlessly changing forms.

Creation occurs through a process of evolution. Alongside the absolute, the transcendence of pure purusha, prakriti rests as potentiality, in a state of apparent nothingness. Out of this most subtle but dynamic state, prakriti evolves, each stage of manifestation progressively more gross or dense until a kind of ladder forms from the Transcendental Self (purusha) to the physical expressions of prakriti in the material world. (Philosophical disputes over the precise workings of this process exist throughout the literature, but they do not concern us here. The general understanding remains constant in all the various interpretations.)

Yoga practice inverses this process. It is evolution in reverse. In yoga, one begins with the physical body and grosser forms of mind and works back through the subtler layers of prakriti to the ultimate source in purusha. Purusha is our true identity—at the core of all manifestation lies the absolute of pure awareness, the true nature of the mind. Vedanta calls this Atman, identical to Brahman, the Ultimate Transcendental Reality. (Atman in the microcosm, Brahman in the macrocosm, but this is only perspective. The Self is everywhere One.) Yoga calls this transcendental reality the purusha, but it is the same thing. The goal of yoga is total realisation of this purusha nature, of pure bliss consciousness—our True Identity. This necessarily involves a detachment from all that is finite, temporal and limited, from all that is prakriti.

In its most subtle form as a state of potentiality, prakriti is the undifferentiated world-ground, a vast but still energy field. Though close to purusha, it remains separate. It exists as creative energy in a state of unmanifest quiet. Here the gunas—the three qualities of energy which comprise prakriti—are at rest in perfect equilibrium. Their stirring into movement and imbalance creates the impetus out of which all matter is shaped. This state of unmanifest quiet is called the Undifferentiate, and out of it three categories of actualisation manifest. The mind is a structure (or function) formed out of the movement of the gunas and containing principles belonging to all three categories.

The Buddhi is the highest principle of the mind. It follows from the first actualisation of the world ground and thus belongs to the first category that arises out of the Undifferentiate, called the Differentiate. Buddhi is the principle of awakening, of intelligence, of cognition. It is the seat of wisdom, which reflects the light of purusha for all it cognises. As the principle of mind closest to purusha, its nature is sattvic: luminous and pure with the reflected radiance of pure consciousness. Because of its proximity to the absolute, its orientation tends to be inwards, towards that reality, rather than outwards into the world. Because of this too, perception at the buddhi level does not identify with content. It is the subtlest and highest form of human awareness. Yet even so, according to Patanjali's absolute dualism, buddhi is still prakriti, insentient in itself and depending upon the light of purusha for all its wisdom.

Following out of the Differentiate, a second level of actualisation occurs, giving rise to the category known as the Unparticularised. Here the individual shape of the mind begins to form, with principles denser than the buddhi, but still more subtle than the ordinary world we recognise with our senses. The principle of asmita or individuation emerges from the unparticularised. As a function of mind it is called the ahamkara. The ahamkara is the "I-maker". Ego identity—that sense of "me" and the "world" as distinct and separate entities—originates here. Ahamkara turns the buddhi away from pure consciousness and towards the manifest world of continually changing forms. Out of this worldly experience, it fabricates the identity called "I"—a false subject or ego. From the unparticularised emerge as well the five tanmatras or sensory potentials. These are the subtle forms of the five ordinary senses.

Finally, out of the Unparticularised, the third level of actualisation occurs, giving rise to the final category called the Particularised. This category includes most of the objects and functions we recognise in the material world. In the arena of the mind, manas emerges. Manas organises sensation. Like a central operator, manas coordinates sensory input with memory and muscular/nervous action. The five karma indriyas (organs of action: hands, feet, mouth, genitals, anus) and the five jnana indriyas (organs of knowledge: sight, hearing, smell, taste, touch) belong to the Particularised as well. The five elements of physical reality manifest here too—ether, air, fire, water and earth. They give rise to all forms in the material world, everything from cows to clouds, from blood to grass, including of course the physical organs of the body out of which the mind principles function.

As these psychic elements interact with the world of experience through time and space, ordinary mind—with its root in ego-consciousness—comes into being. Patanjali sets forth quite a sophisticated psychology. It is a depth psychology (predating Freud by nearly two millennia!) which includes a theory of the unconscious and the definition of various mental states.

It also describes the functional relationship between memory, behaviour and character traits. In this, it is a highly useful psychology that can serve as the theoretical foundation for therapeutic work. As the practice of yoga brings detachment from ego consciousness, a great deal of negative self-material gets released as well. Yoga practice can heal much emotional suffering. Yet yoga is a psychology that never loses sight of the ultimate goal: spiritual transformation. Its vision reaches far beyond the purpose of therapy. Along the path, it may indeed bring positive transformation to the mental states of ordinary life, but its purpose is the ultimate transcendence of ordinary life altogether. The path stops at nothing short of enlightenment itself.

The concept of karma plays a key role in Patanjali's model of the mind. It explains how the conditioned nature of ordinary life comes into being in the first place and how liberation from it can ever occur. Karma refers to action or the fruit of action. It is based upon the principle of cause and effect: all actions have their logical consequences. It is the same in the Biblical maxim, "As you sow, so shall you reap". Yet this concept of karma does not imply determinism. From a particular effect, one can deduce the cause; but from the cause, a particular effect cannot be guaranteed. Too many other—nearly infinite—factors are involved. For instance, if you plant tomato seed, you may or may not get tomatoes. Sunshine, soil, water, insects and birds all may influence the outcome. And these elements too depend upon many influences. But one thing is certain: if you grow tomatoes they did not originate from a tulip bulb.

The working out of karma forms a complex, ever-changing web, as prakriti is never still. It is the nature of the mind (as every yoga practitioner knows!) to be forever busy. Sensory impressions from the external world continually bombard the functions of sight, hearing, smell, taste and touch. And according to Patanjali's epistemology, cognition is possible only because citta is coloured by both the object and the mind itself. As the mind defines the object, so the object defines the mind. Manas then registers the objects of cognition and controls the response. It does so by drawing from the memory bank of karma stored in the mind.

All behaviour leaves its trace in consciousness. These traces are like "grooves" in the mind, where the memory of actions gets laid down, like the sound vibrations that get imprinted into the vinyl of an old-fashioned record. Each time the record is played, the grooves determine the tune that is heard. These mental imprints are called samśkaras in Patanjali's system.

They function as "subliminal activators", memory traces that encourage a repeat of the past action. Sometimes the process is conscious, but more often it is not. In ordinary, conditioned states of consciousness, the mind functions as if on "automatic pilot", encountering experience in the external world and responding according to a known pattern. The repetition of action only serves to deepen the grooves. The traces solidify into tendencies called vasanas. This creates habit energy or the propensity to certain behaviour patterns. The conglomeration of all vasanas forms the karmic deposit (karma-ashaya) of the present life. And this karmic material is like seeds. What has been laid down in the consciousness wants to come to fruition. Throughout life, past karma is in the process of ripening and new karma is being formed by the actions of every day. At death, the reservoir of remaining karma carries over into the next incarnation. This determines the conditions of birth and the circumstances of the next life.

This never-ending cycle is the wheel of samsara, the way of the world, of conditioned existence. It is prakriti dancing. Vedanta calls it maya or delusion. It is delusion because reality gets distorted into a shape determined by personal karma. Habit energy not only ensures the repetition of past action but also determines the kinds of things the senses register. One sees what one is programmed to see. But Patanjali teaches a way off this wheel. It is the practice of Kriya Yoga. Through the two-pronged approach of abhyasa (practice) and vairagya (dispassion), one can understand and transform the workings of one's mind.

Samsara can be transcended. Finally, this psychology is not at all rigid. It is profoundly freeing, in fact, as it culminates in total liberation from the forms of prakriti, in the state called kaivalya. Along the path, it is also freeing, gradually loosening the vasanas and transforming ordinary life. For the evolving mind that begins to awaken through the practice of yoga, it is possible to consciously choose different action, thereby altering the quality of karma being formed. Patanjali calls this the movement from afflicted to non-afflicted thought patterns.

According to Patanjali, five different thought patterns characterise ordinary mental states. These are the vrittis or whirls, the "fluctuations of consciousness" which yoga aims to suspend. Vrittis are the activity of ego-based consciousness. The five vrittis are listed thus: valid-cognition, misconception, imagination, sleep and memory.

Valid-cognition depends upon accurate sense experience. It has three forms: direct perception, inference and reliable testimony. This is the thought pattern of correct knowledge. Of the three, direct perception is the form closest to sensory experience. Here one bites into a fruit and knows through direct sensory contact that it is a peach. Correct knowledge can also derive from inference or the accurate testimony of others. With these, sensory experience is second hand, but still the ultimate source of the valid-cognition. In misconception (the 2nd type of whirl) all this misfires and the result is incorrect knowledge. One incorrectly interprets a sense experience, makes false inference or relies on false testimony. This is the vritti of false knowledge.

With the 3rd whirl, imagination, the process moves inwards to subtler forms of vibration. Here the mind fluctuates with pure conceptualisation, spinning images and fantasies that have no basis in direct sense experience but depend rather upon language. In sleep, the 4th whirl, the process continues with even less connection to direct sense experience. In deep sleep, the mind appears empty, but the experience upon awakening of having slept well or poorly clearly relates to some kind of vritti that had been active during sleep, albeit very subtly. In the 5th whirl, memory, the mind taps into the vasanas or karmic deposits. Of all the vrittis, memory is closest to the unconscious. The store of past actions (from this and maybe even previous lives) feeds the processes of dream, daydream and imagination, supplying raw material in the form of images. Yet memory in itself remains most subtle and deep. These are the whirls most difficult to suspend.

Through meditation, the yogi strives to modify, control or suspend these five types of vrittis. If this state can be maintained, it leads to samprajnata samadhi, the lower form of samadhi, known as object-oriented ecstasy. It is called "object-oriented" because some vrittis remain. Though the vrittis of ordinary consciousness are suspended, sattvic vrittis are present—radiant and pure and whispering of purusha. Not until asamprajnata samadhi, which is "objectless" or without vrittis of any kind, is the goal of yoga reached. However, in the lower states of samadhi, sattvic mind can make for a very blissful existence. Though vrittis still occur, they are no longer afflicted. It is these non-afflicted vrittis that provide the yogi with the momentum to reach full samadhi. These positive thought waves have great benefit, as they facilitate the process of yoga.

It is through the mind that the mind is set free. The sattvic vrittis of samprajnata samadhi enhance the desire for total liberation. And right action follows, the kind of behaviour that leads towards the ultimate transcendence of all vrittis. It is important to distinguish between afflicted and non-afflicted vrittis. And each of the five types of vrittis, in principle, can be either afflicted or non-afflicted. Afflicted vrittis perpetuate the wheel of samsara. Non-afflicted vrittis contain the seeds for the transcendence of all vrittis. They infuse everyday life with a high degree of sattvic energy and culminate in their own cessation.

So what causes the ordinary vrittis of the mind? What are the factors that keep one bound in conditioned existence? Here in a sense is the heart of Patanjali's psychology. Human suffering arises out of ordinary consciousness itself, Patanjali explains, where attachment to the forms of prakriti obscures the true reality—purusha. Patanjali identifies five qualities of mind that create and maintain these vrittis of ordinary consciousness. They are called the five kleshas or sources of affliction. They are the root cause of the "misidentification with the modifications of the mind" which yoga practice aims to eradicate.

Avidya is the first klesha. It is the source of all the others. Translated often as ignorance, but implying much more, avidya is the opposite of vidya, which means seeing. True sight sees the truth, and that is vidya. True sight means realising Ultimate Reality. Its opposite, avidya, is thus a most severe type of blindness. Avidya is spiritual ignorance, the greatest and most fundamental cause of suffering. All the other sources of affliction derive from avidya. Yoga practice aims to transform avidya into vidya. This is what "yoga chittas vrittis nirodha" indicates.

Asmita, the second klesha, derives directly from avidya. Asmita is the formation of ego-identity. This is the ahamkara function of the mind, which understands all reality in terms of itself. Because of avidya, the mind identifies with its own particulars. It forms a "self" out of the physical body, the fluctuating content of the mind, and the store of karma and memory. Identity can extend beyond into possessions, associations and all the particulars of a certain life. These things that are relative, changing and finite become reified into a self, obscuring the true Self.

Raga and dvesa are the third and fourth kleshas, attachment and aversion. Together, these two factors help create and maintain the ego-identity. Attachment and aversion are like the two antennae of ordinary consciousness. The ego encounters everything in the world in these terms: either good for me (attraction) or bad for me (aversion). All meaning and worth of the thing encountered derives from its reference to the ego-identity. I like someone because he is useful to me, dislike someone because he offends me... Most of which does not fit into either category gets ignored. The ego does not usually register that which is irrelevant to its interest. Most awareness thus centres round this fabricated identity, the ego. Attraction and aversion help solidify its form, as in "I am a person who loves dogs and horses... or I am a person who hates action films and black coffee..." Abhinivesa is the fifth klesha. This final cause of suffering is the will-to-live. More precisely, it is a clinging to the life that the ego understands or the fear of death. It includes a strong attachment to the false self's activity of attraction and aversion and a deep fear of the dissolution of this fabricated identity. Thus, it can imply both a fear of literal death as well as a resistance to the process of yoga. For yoga practice strives to undo the false identity. With abhinivesa, one clings to the vrittis of ordinary consiousness and lacks faith or trust in anything more. Here one is truly "stuck". Even though ordinary consciousness cannot realise purusha, it can still trust that greater reality is possible. Without the faith that something more is possible, how can one strive to attain it?

An answer can be found in Patanjali. It is called Kriya Yoga—a method of mind transformation that undermines the hold of the kleshas. Through this yoga—and all the particulars of abhyasa (practice) and vairagya (dispassion)—the yogi strives to eradicate the kleshas and dissolve the mind into its purusha nature. This is what yoga is about, and what the Yoga Sutra defines so methodically. As yoga practice involves the movement from afflicted to non-afflicted vrittis, it can bring much healing, both to the individual yogi and to this suffering world. But the practice does not end there. It is not until the end of all vrittis—in the state of ultimate liberation called kaivalya—that yoga reaches it final purpose. The mind is an instrument programmed to contain the seed of its own transcendence. For the ultimate goal is always beyond the mind in pure purusha awareness.

Whether it is possible to reach this state and still be alive in a body is an interesting question. How can a mind and body function without "thought-waves"? Is the goal the total cessation of vrittis (death?) or the cessation of misidentification with these "thought-waves" (death of ego-consciousness)? These questions make the study of the Sanskrit texts a fascinating quest. In classical yoga, the body drops away soon after complete enlightenment. Vedanta recognises the state of jivan-mukta, enlightenment in this life. Yet despite these different understandings, the path of practice remains the same. And perhaps at some point of awareness even these distinctions disappear, as if "life" and "death" are mere categories of samsara and enlightenment lies beyond them both, in a state the rational mind could never grasp. "Human kind cannot bear very much reality." But yoga is not complete until that Ultimate Reality subsumes everything.

YOUR BRAIN ON TRAUMA

So how exactly do yoga asanas and pranayama quell agitation or energize a collapsed spirit? Before we talk more specifics, a little neurophysiology lesson is in order. Under normal conditions, the body is hardwired to protect us from danger or stressful situations; trouble ensues when its process is interrupted. The best way to understand the human response is to look at animals in the wild. Sounds a bit far-fetched, perhaps, but Levine contends that our nervous system has a lot more in common with our four-hoofed brethren than we might think. A group of deer grazing in a meadow, for example, may appear happy-go-lucky, but they are continually on the lookout for predators lurking in the forest nearby. The very first thing the deer do when they perceive danger is to stop, stay very still, and listen. This hyper-vigilant stage of arrest activates the sympathetic nervous system (in charge of the fight-or-flight response to danger) and serves two purposes. One, it allows them to figure out what the threat might be and where it's coming from (a smell in the air or a rustle in the bushes), and two, it helps them be more invisible to a predator. The moment the deer feel a predator's presence, they take flight, running to safety as fast as they can. If one falters and the coyote catches up to her, her first instinct is to rise up and fight back. If that fails, and she gets caught, she freezes, her muscles stiffening against the assault, and then folds, going limp and numb-helpless to protect herself.

The fold or collapse state of hypo-arousal activates the parasympathetic nervous system, shutting down the body's defences, allowing her to dissociate from the event, and preventing her from feeling too much pain. If she's able to fool her predator and race to safety, she'll tremble, literally shaking off the event, and return to the meadow in time for the next meal. While her brain registers the event and files away a "do not go near those bushes on the right" message, her ordeal is over and done with.

The human nervous system works much the same way. When we perceive danger, the sympathetic nervous system and the hypothalamic-pituitary-adrenal (HPA) axis mobilize the body's fight-or-flight resources.

Stress hormones pour into the bloodstream so we can react appropriately. They increase our heart rate, divert blood into our large muscle groups (arms and legs), and speed up reaction time. An increase in cortisol releases sugar as fuel into the bloodstream so we can think and move faster. In the meantime, the HPA axis communicates with the rest of the body, instructing the digestive, reproductive, and immune systems to slow down and wait out the danger.

All this activity creates a state of hyper-arousal and fuels the emotions and actions we need to first gain sensory information and then either fight an aggressor (anger) or, if need be, flee the scene to safety (anxiety and fear). Just like our animal friends, humans can also experience complete collapse, or hypo-arousal-when the parasympathetic nervous system activates to help us survive horrific acts of violence. Both the alert and the fold states are designed to be short-lived, functioning to keep us alive and safe from harm.

Yoga mitigates the fight-or-flight response through a combination of active asanas, pranayama, and deep relaxation. As we can see, our autonomic nervous system was designed to be on the lookout for danger and keep us safe. Problems arise when the pain and traumatic residue, or samskara, remains in the body long after the event is over and the brain cannot discriminate between what is in the past and what is a real, present threat. The body's posture (rigid or collapsed) continues to signal danger, so the nervous system goes in search of the perpetrator, assigning blame wherever it can. Levine says, "If frightening sensations are not given the time and attention they need to move through the body and resolve or dissolve, the individual will continue to be gripped by fear."

Calm the Waters

In addition to the recently concluded NIH study, other studies and plenty of anecdotal evidence support the claim that yoga mitigates the fight-or-flight response through a combination of active asanas, pranayama (with particular emphasis on the exhalation), and deep relaxation. It does this by decreasing the sympathetic nervous system's reactive response and increasing the parasympathetic relaxation response. Jay P., an Air Force vet from the Boston area, who experienced a brutal assault when he was stationed overseas in the early '80s-too horrible for him even to describe-shares a story that perfectly demonstrates yoga's calming effect.

One manifestation of Jay's trauma is acute anxiety, which gets triggered when he's in a crowd of people. After a particularly difficult therapy session, he says, "I was feeling a lot worse than when I came in." He got to the metro station in Boston, right in the middle of rush hour. His anxiety built as the crowd grew bigger; at one point, he says, "I felt like, 'I don't think I can do this.'"

Feeling quite agitated, he turned around to leave, and then he saw a woman standing nearby holding a little child. "I put my hand on my belly and started to breathe-really focusing and paying attention to my breathing as I looked at the little kid and her mom." Suddenly the crowd and Jay's anxiety seemed to dissipate-everything felt more manageable. "I had put myself into a shavasana-type pose with a sweet little kid in front of me," he says, and it worked.

Re-energize the Body

Less well known is yoga's ability to put the brakes on an overly active parasympathetic nervous system (PNS). Recognized for its role in the relaxation response, the PNS can also get stuck on unhealthy overdrive. As our animal friends demonstrated, the freeze-and-fold response involves shutting down the body's responses and lowering blood pressure and heart rate, all of which allows a victim to dissociate from the traumatic event, and prevents him from feeling too much pain.

Unfortunately for trauma survivors, long after the event has passed, they may still feel numb and depressed, constantly tired, and completely dissociated from their feelings. Levine says chronic immobility paralyzes a trauma victim, and fear of unleashing her feelings deepens her sense of paralysis. It's important, he says, for survivors to learn to disentangle the fear and helplessness from their immobility.

Seleni (again a pseudonym), who grew up in an African country that has experienced a great deal of violence, was trafficked into domestic servitude in the United States. Scooped up into the arms of Project Reach, a programme that serves survivors of human trafficking, Seleni learned that she would be required to repeatedly tell (and hence relive) her story-to prosecutors, lawyers, judges, and therapists-in hopes of identifying and eventually prosecuting her abusers. Hopper, programme director of Project Reach, says she sat with Seleni, watching and listening as she recounted the horrific details of her plight. At one point, Hopper noticed that Seleni's body began to sag forward, growing heavier and weaker until it gave way, and her head and upper body collapsed on the desk in front of her. She told Hopper that she shuts down this way when she has to talk about her ordeal; and when that happens, she knows she won't be able sleep that night.

Instead of continuing with the story, Hopper asked Seleni to stand up. They breathed together-emphasizing the inhalation-gently energizing Seleni's body and activating her sympathetic nervous system. In a slow, rhythmic way, Hopper led Seleni through a dynamic mountain pose, encouraging her to move between a posture in which she collapses (shoulders hunched forward, neck and head bowed) and one in which she lifts her chest, elongates her spine, and raises her head up. Seleni's inhalation deepened and she began to coordinate arm movements with the rise and fall of her breath. When she returned to her chair, Seleni sat up straighter and her face brightened. She even shared a few spiritual songs from her tradition that always made her feel better.

ENGAGE THE MIND

Meditation can also help trauma victims to bring their nervous system back into balance. But sitting in silent meditation, with just their thoughts to keep them company, can be terrifying, according to van der Kolk. He says trauma-sensitive people "have their sense of time thrown off and think something will last forever." So he suggests those with PTSD get more comfortable with postures and breath work and learn relaxation techniques before moving on to meditation. Mantra meditation and yoga nidra provide two alternatives to following one's thoughts in silence. Using a mantra gives the mind an anchor, a companion on the journey inward, something to return to as memories and sensations surface and dissolve. Yoga nidra or Richard Miller's iRest practice helps them stay present to what's going on-feeling the energy of the body, and exploring sensations without judgement or attachment.

While no one we spoke with believes yoga alone has the power to heal the pain trauma survivors endure, every single survivor, teacher, and expert wholeheartedly believes yoga provides a powerful ally on the journey home, and allows survivors-many for the very first time-to create a loving and nurturing relationship with their bodies. We can't predict or control what the future holds, nor can we change what the past has dealt, but we can learn to care deeply about ourselves and to embrace the present.

CHAPTER

8

Bhakti Yoga Sadhana

God is the silent witness of your thoughts; He is the internal leader of your heart and mind. You cannot hide anything from Him. Become guileless and straightforward. A devotee of Hari is always meek and humble. Name of God "Hari" is always on his lips. He sheds profuse tears when he is alone. He is very pious. He is friendly towards all. He has equal-vision. He does well always. He never hurts the feelings of others. He has a spotless character. He never covets the property of others. He sees Hari in all beings.

Bhakti can move mountains. Nothing is impossible to it. It was the devotion of Mira that converted a snake into a flower garland, poison into nectar and a bed of nails into a bed of roses. It was the devotion of Prahlada that turned fire into ice. A devotee should become an embodiment of goodness. He must be ever ready to do well to living beings. That devotee who is intent upon the welfare of all beings obtains the peace of the Eternal. He, who rejoices in the welfare of all, gets the Darshan of the Lord. He develops Advaitic consciousness eventually.

Repetition of God's name, Satsanga, singing His name, Service of Bhagavatas, study of the Bhagavata or the Ramayana, living in Brindavan, Pandharpur, Chitrakuta or Ayodhya, are the six means for developing Bhakti. Anger and lust are the two inner enemies that stand in the way of developing Bhakti. From lust follow the ten vices that are mentioned in Manusamhita—love of hunting, gambling, sleeping by day, slandering, company with bad women, drinking, singing love-songs, vulgar music, dancing, aimlessly wandering about. Anger begets eight kinds of vices. All evil qualities proceed from anger. If you can eradicate anger, all bad qualities will die of them. The eight vices are: Injustice, rashness, persecution, jealousy, taking possession of others' property, harsh words and cruelty.

How are Bhaktas to be known? Lord Krishna has given a description of them. You will find it in Bhagavatam. "They do not care for anything. Their hearts are fixed on Me. They are very humble. They have equal vision. They have no attachment towards anybody or anything. They are without 'mine-ness'. They have no egoism. They make no distinction between sorrow and happiness. They do not take anything from others. They can bear heat, cold and pain. They have love for all living beings. They have no enemy. They are serene. They possess exemplary character."

At this point is a Sadhana for advanced students. This is highly useful for getting quick, solid progress in the spiritual path. Get up at 4 a.m. Start your Japa on any Asana you have mastered. Do not take food or drink for 14 hours. Do not get up from the Asana. Control passing urine till sunset if you can manage. Finish the Japa at sunset. Take milk and fruits after sunset. Householders can practise this during holidays. Practise this once a fortnight or once a month or once weekly.

There are one more Sadhana for 10 days. You can do this while the Christmas holidays or Puja holidays or summer vacation. Shut yourself in an airy room. Do not talk to anybody. Do not see anybody. Do not hear anything. Get up at 4 a.m. Start Japa of the Mantra of your Ishta Devata or your Guru Mantra and finish it at sunset. Afterward take some milk and fruits or Kheer (milk and rice boiled with sugar). Take rest for one or two hours. But continue the Japa. Then again start the Japa seriously. Retire to bed at 11 in the night. You can combine meditation along with Japa. Make all arrangements for bath, food, etc., inside the room. Have two rooms if you can manage, one for bath and one for meditation. Repeat this four times a day. This practice can be kept up even for 40 days. You will have wonderful result and various experiences. You will enter into Samadhi. You will have Darshan of your Ishtam. I assure you.

There is a Anushthana for 40 days. You will have to do Japa of Rama Mantra one Lakh and twenty five thousand times in the following manner for 40 days, at the rate of 3000 daily. During the last five days do 4000 daily. Get up at 4. A.m. Write down in a thin paper 'Rama, Rama' 300 times. Then cut it into small pieces. Each piece will contain one Rama Nama. Then roll it with a small ball of Atta (wheat flour paste). Writing will take two or three hours according to your strength and capacity. Then you will have to cut one by one. You will have to do the whole process by sitting on one Asana. If you find it difficult to sit on one Asana, you can have change of Asana. But you should not leave your seat. Some use a special ink made of saffron, musk, camphor, etc., and special writing pen made up of a sharp-pointed thin, Tulasi-stick. You can use ordinary ink and pen if you cannot get the above special ink and special pen. You will have to do the Anushthana on the banks of Ganga, Yamuna, Godavari, Kaveri or Narmada, at Rishikesh, Benares, Hardwar, or Prayag. You can do it at home, if you find it difficult to move to these places. Take milk and fruits and Palahar during these days. Two Punjabis, a student of law, and his father, are having this Anushthana in Rishikesh. Throw the balls in the Ganga or any river for fishes. You will develop wonderful patience. You will get Divine Grace.

Lear the whole of the Ramayana 108 times with purity and concentration. This can be done within three years if you can devote three hours daily. You can go through the book three times in a month. You will acquire Siddhis. You will have Darshan of Lord Rama.

Bhakti Yoga and Jnana Yoga are not incompatibles like acids and alkalis. One can combine Ananya Bhakti (one-pointed devotion) with Jnana Yoga. The fruit of Bhakti Yoga is Jnana. Highest love (Para Bhakti and Jnana are one. Perfect knowledge is love. Perfect love is knowledge. Sri Sankara, the Advaita Kevala Jnani, was a great Bhakta of Lord Hari, Hara and Devi. Jnana Deva of Alandi, Poona, a great Yogi of late, was a Bhakta of Lord Krishna. Sri Ramakrishna Paramahamsa worshipped Kali and got Jnana through Swami Totapuri, his Advaita Guru.

God Chaitanya was a fine Advaita Vedantic Scholar, and yet he danced in streets and market places, singing Hari's names. Appaya Dikshitar, a famous Jnani of Adaipalam, North Arcot District, Madras, the author of Siddhanta Lesha and various other Vedantic books was a devotee of Lord Siva. It behoves, therefore, that Bhakti can be combined with much advantage with Jnana.

May we hear with our ears and see with our eyes nothing but what is pure, so that with our senses unperturbed, remembering God, meditating on Him, singing His praise and repeating His name, we may attain life as that of the Gods. Om Santi.

Kirtan At Home

Kirtan is an easy way for attaining God-consciousness. At night all the members of the house should sit in a circle and do Kirtan for one hour before the picture of Lord Krishna. The servants of the house also should be included. Sing any Name of the Lord as Siva, Hare Ram, Sita Ram, Raghupati Raghava Rajaram, etc., in a chorus with one Svara, Tala harmoniously. Nada Brahman will be generated. You will forget the body and the world and enter into ecstatic state. Practise, try and feel yourself. Mere tall talk will not do. Just as the intoxication that you get by taking a dose of opium lasts for hours, the Divine intoxication that you get from Kirtan will last for some hours during the following day also. At night you will be free from bad dreams. During Kirtan a special spiritual wave comes from the indweller of your heart and purifies the mind and Pranamaya Kosha. All diseases are cured thereby. Doctor's bills are saved. Sattva flows from the Lord to your mind, just as oil flows from one vessel to another vessel. Kirtan gives you strength to face the difficulties in the battle of life. Singing the Names of the Lord is a mental tonic.

Evening Katha At Home

Four people can join together and read regularly the Bhagavad Gita, the Ramayana or the Bhagavata in the evening or and suitable time. Svadhyaya or study of Holy Scriptures is Kriya Yoga. It is of immense benefit for householders who do not find much time for serious spiritual practices and constant meditation. The study itself is a form of meditation. When the mind is concentrated on Divine thoughts, it is filled with purity. The gross mind is rendered subtle.

What Should Ladies Do

In India, religion is maintained by the ladies only. There is peculiar religious instinct in them. Hindu ladies are highly devotional. They infuse the religious spirit in the males through their daily conduct and practical life. They get up in the early morning, wash the house, take bath, do Japa, make a small temple in their house and keep their pictures of the Lord and Pooja vessels, etc. They keep the place sacred and in the evening do Arati and prayer. The atheistic male members of the house are forced to do some prayer or other through their influence, Because of fear. In reality the ladies of the house govern the house. They are the manifestations of Sakti. The husband is not entitled to do any religious rite without her presence by his side.

"Yatra naryastu pujyante ramante tatra devatah,
Yatrai tastu na pujyante sarvastatraphalah kriyah"

—Manu Smriti III-56.

"Where women are honored, there Devas are pleased; but where they are not honoured, there no sacred rite is fruitful." Such is the glory of Hindu ladies. My earnest prayer is that they should sing the Name of the Lord in the early morning as soon as they get up. They should train their children also to sing the Names. The whole house will be charged with spiritual vibrations. Even when they cook and draw water from the wells, they should be singing in mild tone the Names of the Lord. A strong habit of repeating the Names of the Lord will be formed in two months. This it is quite sufficient for attaining God-consciousness. Singing the Names of the Lord is a extremely simple method for getting Darshan of the Lord in this Kali-Yuga. Even when anyone dies, the habit of singing the Name of the Lord will come to his rescue.

Duties Of Womanhood

Since time immemorial Sita, Savitri, Damayanti, Nalayani, Anasuya and Draupadi have been regarded as sacred ideals of Indian Womanhood. They are sublime and exemplary characters who have exalted womanhood to the height of divine perfection.

Modern women should draw inspiration from their lives and try to tread their path. On condition that such characters continue to exercise their influence upon the lives and character of Indian ladies, so long they will be looked upon with admiration and reverence by their sisters of other countries.

All of them were subjected to very severe tests in which their purity, courage, patience and other virtues were put to and nobly did they come out through those tests. Hindu women are, since the dawn of the early civilisation, distinguished for their disinterested love and self-abnegation.

What a wife is to a Hindu husband is well illustrated by a verse in the Ramayana where Sri Rama referred to Sita says:

Karyeshu Mantree, Karaneshu Dasee,

Dharmeshu Patnee, Kshamaya Dharitree,

Sneheshu Mata, Sayaneshu Rambha,

Rangecha Sakhi, Lakshmana Sa Priya Me.

"In counsel she is my counselor, in action she is my servant, in spiritual performances she is my partner, in tolerance she is like the earth, in affection she is like unto my mother, in bed she is like the celestial Rambha and in play she is my companion. Such certainly, O Lakshmana, is my beloved..." This is the Hindu ideal of a wife.

The everlasting fidelity of a Hindu woman to her husband makes her an ideal of the feminine world. It makes her sublime and lofty. This sublime virtue still runs deep in the heart of hearts of every Hindu woman of India superior to any of the other countries in national integrity and honour.

The inspirational strength of the home is woman. The home is the origin and the beginning of every form of social organization. It is the nursery of the nation. It is the sweet place or centre wherein children are trained for future citizenship. The woman illumines the home through the glory of motherhood. Man is powerless of doing the domestic duties incident upon the rearing up of the children. Right conduct, Good habits, formation of character is created in children spontaneously in a well-regulated home under the personal influence of the mother. The loving kindness and the cultured gentleness of the mother help the children to unfold their native talents and dormant capacities quickly. Children absorb ideas by suggestion and imitation. Early training and impressions are lasting formation of character can be done by efficiently by mothers at home. Therefore, home is the beautiful training ground for the building up of character in children under the personal guidance of the mother.

Women are the bedrock or backbone or the basis for sustaining religion and national strength and prosperity. There is no dissimilarity between her and Lakshmi, the Goddess of Beauty, Grace and Prosperity. Manu says, "That woman who does always good, who is efficient in work, sweet in speech, devoted to her Dharmas and service to her husband, is really no human being but a Goddess." If the mother trains her children on the right lines she is rendering a great service indeed to the nation and the national culture.

Women have got ample opportunities to increase and improve and the prosperity and national health. They actually build the nation. They can utilize their talents and abilities in making the home the cradle of culture character, personal ability and religious upheaval. It is therefore wrong to say that their life is cramped or stunted by attending to the duties at home and that no scope is given for evolution and freedom. This is a sad mistake indeed! The life of a woman is as noble and serious as that of a man. There is no doubt of this.

It is the women that keep up the life and happiness of the home through their smile, charming personality, grace, tender affection, sweet speech and angelic presence. The home will be a real void without them. It will lose its peculiar charm and beauty without their presence.

It will be of enormous benefit to know what the Great Ones have said about the ideal of conduct and deportment that a woman should try to live up to. Sri Rama instructs Kausalya, his mother, as follows: "To a woman so long as she is alive, the husband is indeed the Lord and God. That woman, who, though noblest of all and given to the practice of vows and fasts, does not look after her husband, will indeed obtain an unmeritorious future. Even if a woman has never bowed to the Gods and has ceased to worship them, she obtains the highest heaven by serving her husband. A woman should be absorbed in the service of her husband, taking delight in his pleasure and his good. This is the path of the Dharma, known for long ages, revealed in the Vedas, and remembered by the world. There is nothing more cruel for a woman than to desert her husband. To attend upon and to serve one's husband is no doubt the highest duty of a woman. So long as a woman lives, her husband is her only master."

Afterward again there is Kanva Rishi's advice to Sakuntala on the eve of her departure from his Ashram to King Dushyanta's residence. Kanva Rishi says: "Sakuntala! Serve all your elders. Though your Lord is angry with you at times, do not go against his wishes. Do not be too much attached in enjoyment. Treat your dependants and co-wives with motherly affection and tenderness. Be an affectionate companion to your sisters-in-law. Be obedient to your mother-in-law. These attributes will make you the true mistress of the house. Otherwise, you will give pain and trouble to the whole family."

It is the responsibility of the lady of the house to get up before her husband in the early hours of the dawn, take her bath and perform the household work. Tiruvalluvar's wife shampooed the feet of her husband, sleep after her husband and rose up in the morning before he got up from bed. She is regarded as a model woman.

To a lady the husband is really the highest ornament of all ornaments. Being separated from him, she, conversely beautiful, does not shine.

The Hindu scriptures say that the wife must be very obedient and that the husband is God to her. Some unaware persons take advantage of this and exercise undue power over their wives and keep them under extreme subordination. Is this not a sad mistake? The personal influence of women at home is essential to unify the various interests of the family. It is women alone who can rear and nurse children. Hindu wives are queens in their own homes. Woman is in no way inferior to man. The home is a co-operative organization. It flourishes on the principle of division of labor. The husband should not think that he is superior to his wife, simply because he is the earning member of the family. Women have a definite field of their own. They are mothers of the house. The extraordinary abilities and intellectual attainments, and the magnetic personality of the modern women are a standing monument to their undoubted equality with men. The husbands should treat their wives with intense love and respect. They should be regarded as equals in all respects and be held in the light of partners in life. Manu says, "The householder should first serve his relatives and dependants with food and then take the remaining food along with his wife," hinting thereby at the position of equal footing on which she is to be treated. If a man earns and the wife stays at home, it does not mean that the woman is a parasite and a slave. She is indeed the builder of the nation. Verily, women exercise an authority over their husbands through their love, tenderness, affection, grace, beauty, selfless service and fidelity, purity and self-abnegation.

In the European country the woman is wife. In India the woman is the mother. Mother is worshipped. Mother is considered as the Goddess Lakshmi of the house. The Srutis emphatically declare, "Let thy mother be thy God." The late Ashutosh Mukherji, Vice-Chancellor of the Calcutta University used to wash the feet of his mother and drink the water before he went to his office. This water is called 'Charanamrit'. It is a great purifier of the heart. In the West the wife governs the home. In an Indian home the mother rules. In the West the mother has to be subordinate to the wife. In India the wife has to be subordinate to the mother.

If woman be pure she can save and purify man. Woman can purify the race. Woman can make a home a sacred temple. The Hindu women have been the custodians of the Hindu race. The Hindu religion, the Hindu culture and civilization still survive in spite of the many foreign invasions, when other civilizations have come and gone, on account of the purity of the Hindu women. The women are taught to regard chastity as their most priceless possession, and the loss of it as equal to the eternal damnation of their souls. Religion is ingrained in the Hindu women from their very childhood. Hindu women illumine and enliven the house through the glory of their purity. This is the secret of the endurance of the Hindu religion, civilisation and culture.

Advice To Householders

Begin that pure life of a Yogi the very day on which you read these lines. No leniency to mind. Self-reliance is indispensably requisite. You can get suggestions from outside. But you will have to tread the path yourself, to place each step yourself in the spiritual ladder.

You will have to train your wife also. She also will have to do rigid Sadhana. Mere gossiping will not do. If she serves the husband nicely and takes care of his body with the right mental attitude and gives him the wants of the flesh, food and drinks as soon as he comes down from meditation, she can have Self-realisation in and through the form of her husband alone, like Laila in Majnu, Savitri in Satyavan, Anasuya in Atri.

That house is a miserable place, veritable hell on earth wherein the husband moves up in spirituality and the wife pulls him down in sensual grooves and vice versa. They should be harmoniously blended or joined by the thread of the knowledge of the Self, each aspiring eagerly for attaining God-consciousness.

That house is really a Vaikuntha where the husband and wife lead an ideal Divine Life, singing Hari's Name, repeating His Mantra 200 Malas daily, and studying the Ramayana and the Bhagavata, controlling the Indriyas and serving Bhaktas and Sannyasins.

Renunciation is mental, it brings peace. There is no loss in renunciation. You renounce the illusory sense happiness to get the Supreme, Eternal Bliss and Immortality. Stand this in mind. Do not be guided and influenced by public opinion. March boldly and cheerfully in the path of Truth, consulting your inner conscience and hearing the inner, small, shrill, sweet voice of the soul. Do not be hasty in doing any outward renunciation. The world is the best teacher. Unfold the Divinity by remaining in the world alone. Nivritti Marga is extremely difficult. Ninety per cent fail in this path.

Save as much money as much possible. Do 200 Malas of Japa. Cut off society. Keep company with one Sattvic man. Spend every second profitably. Serve sick people. Share what you have a small portion with poor people.

May the Divine Glory shine in your face!

Nil Desperandum

Sin is a fault committed by the ignorant Jiva during his journey towards Sat-Chit-Ananda abode. Once you make up your mind to tread the path of truth all sins will be destroyed. Lord Krishna gives His assurance: "Even if the most sinful worship me, with undivided heart, he too must be accounted righteous for he hath rightly resolved. Speedily he becometh dutiful and goeth to eternal peace. Know thou for certain that My devotee never perisheth." When such is the power of the inverse name (Mara, Mara), what to speak of the glory of repeating Rama, Rama with Bhava from the bottom of the heart! Ajamila who was in a degraded and abject state on account of his bad character attained Mukti by repeating 'Narayana' once in his death-bed by calling his son by his name Narayana. Licentious Vemanna of Andhra Desa became a full-blown Yogi by his devotion to mother Kali. Grieve not, my dear friends. Fear not. Stand up. Gird up the loins. Fight with the Indriyas and Vasanas. Become a Yogi. Forget the past. A glorious, brilliant future is awaiting you. Cheer up yourself. Purify. Concentrate. Do Japa and Kirtan. Meditate. Realise the Sat-Chit-Ananda Atman!

BHAKTI YOGA

Bhakti yoga is a spiritual path or spiritual practice within Hinduism focused on the cultivation of love and devotion towards God. It has been defined as a practice of devotion towards God, solely motivated by the sincere, loving desire to please God, rather than the hope of divine reward or the fear of divine punishment. It is a means towards a state of spiritual liberation or enlightenment through the "realisation", or the attainment of "oneness" with God. *Bhakti yoga* is often considered by Hindus to be the easiest way for ordinary people to attain such a spiritually liberated state, because although it is a form of *yoga*, its practice is not as rigorous as most other yogic schools, and it is possible to practice *bhakti yoga* without needing to become a full-time yogi.

The origins of Bhakti can be seen in the upanishads, specifically the Shvetashvatara Upanishad. The *Bhagavad Gita*, and the *Puranas* are important scriptures that expound the philosophy of *bhakti yoga*. Hindu movements in which *bhakti yoga* is the main practice are called *bhakti* movements - the major schools of which are Vaishnavism, Shaivism, and Shaktism.

Philosophy

Bhakti is a Sanskrit term that signifies an attitude of devotion to a personal God which is similar to a number of interpersonal relationships between humans, such as between lovers or friends. The difference is that in *bhakti*, the relationship is between a soul (that of the devotee) and a "supersoul" (God). *Bhakti* is a yogic path, in that the devotee's aim is of loving union with God. While the exact form (deity) through which God is worshiped and the exact nature of the union varies between different schools, the essence of the practice displays remarkable homogeneity.

The *Bhagavata Purana* teaches nine primary forms of *bhakti*, as explained by Prahlada:

- *sravana* ("listening" to the scriptural stories of Krishna and his companions),
- *kîrtana* ("praising"; this usually refers to ecstatic group singing),
- *visnoh smarana* ("remembering" or fixing the mind on Vishnu),
- *pâda-sevana* (rendering service),
- *arcana* (worshiping an image),

- *vandana* (paying homage),
- *dâsya* (servitude),
- *sâkhya* (friendship), and
- *âtma-nivedana* (complete surrender of the self). *(From* Bhagavata Purana, *7.5.23-24.)*

These nine principles of devotional service are described as helping the devotee remain constantly in touch with God. The processes of *japa* and internal meditation on the aspirant devotee's *ista-devatâ,* or chosen deity, are especially popular in most *bhakti yoga* schools. The Indians spiritual teacher Meher Baba stated "Out of a number of practices which lead to the ultimate goal of humanity - God-Realisation - *Bhakti Yoga* is one of the most important. Almost the whole of humanity is concerned with *Bhakti Yoga,* which, in simple words, means the art of worship. But it must be understood in all its true aspects, and not merely in a narrow and shallow sense, in which the term is commonly used and interpreted. The profound worship based on the high ideals of philosophy and spirituality, prompted by divine love, doubtless constitutes true *Bhakti Yoga.*

The Bhagavad Gita

The *Bhagavad Gita* is a cornerstone of Hindu *bhakti* theism, especially among Vaishnavists. The *Bhagavad Gita* stresses that love and innocent pure intentions are the most powerful motive forces in a devotee's spiritual life.

- Engage your mind always in thinking of Me, become My devotee, offer obeisances to Me and worship Me. Being completely absorbed in Me, surely you will come to Me. *(B-Gita 9.34)*
- One can understand Me as I am, as the Supreme Personality of Godhead, only by devotional service. And when one is in full consciousness of Me by such devotion, he can enter into the kingdom of God. *(B-Gita 18.55)*

Branches

There are three main groups of *bhakti yoga* practitioners in Hinduism: the Shaivists who worship Shiva and his family, including Ganesh and Murugan; the Vaishnavists, who worship Vishnu and his avatars such as Krishna and Rama; and the Shaktists, who primarily worship *Devis*, such as Durga, Kali, Lakshmi and Parvati.

All these groups have great respect for the others' primary deities, while considering their own paramount in their worship. Although each deity is perceived from a human perspective as having a slightly different form and somewhat different primary and secondary qualities, the most advanced practitioners in each group, as well as the scriptures of each group, believe that each deity is substantively intertwined with all the others in such a way that, essentially, they are all the same being: a single transcendent God.

Notable Proponents of Bhakti

- Narada Muni
- Hanuman
- The Alvars c. 2nd century to 8th century
- The Nayanars 5th century to 1010 century
- Adi Shankara 788 to 820
- Natamuni c 10th century
- Alavandar (Yamuna) 916 to 1036
- Ramanujacharya 1017 to 1137
- Madhvacharya 1238 to 1317
- Vedanta Desika 1268 to 1370
- Jayadeva 12th century
- Nimbarka 13th century
- Annamacharya 1408 to 1503
- Vallabha Acharya 1479 to 1531
- Chaitanya Mahaprabhu 1486 to 1533
- Poonthanam 1547 to 1640

- Bhadrachala Ramadasu (Kancherla Gopanna) c. 1620 to 1680
- Guru Ravidass
- Narsinh Mehta
- Meera
- Swami Ramanand 1738 to 1802
- Swaminarayan 1781 to 1830
- Tyâgarâja died 1847
- Bhaktivinoda Thakur 1838 to 1914
- Sai Baba of Shirdi 1838 to 1918
- Ramana Maharshi 1878 to 1950
- Bhaktivedanta Swami Prabhupada 1896 to 1977
- Pramukh Swami Maharaj 1921
- Jagadguru Kripalu Maharaj 1922
- Srila Bhaktivedanta Narayana Goswami Maharaja 1921-2010

CHAPTER

9

Patanjali's Kriya Yoga

Patanjali also presented a version of kriya yoga, the path of transmutative action (*i.e.*, the act of changing into a higher form) in his Yoga Sutra. Kriya yoga can best be described as a form of internal karma yoga. That is, by perfecting the niyamas or self-disciplines of Patanjali's eight-limbed path, particularly tapas (austerity), svadhyaya (self-study), and isvara pranidhana (devotion to the Lord), a yogi erases Samskara (subliminal activators) from his subconscious. Samskaras are like karma scars that result from good or bad behaviour. They are indelible memories, imprinted on the subconscious, that propel the conscious mind to act; they are what dictate a person's birth, life experiences, and death.

These activators cause the constant chatter or fluctuations in the mind that separate a person from purusha and make it impossible for him to experience it. An individual has good kinds of samskara and bad kinds, according to the Yoga Sutra. The bad kind keep the conscious mind actively seeking experience outside itself, regardless of whether that experience is pleasurable or painful. The good kind stop the conscious mind from seeking and attaching itself to external objects and senses. The resultant cessation (nirodhah) of vritti (fluctuations) and samskara brings true liberation.

The Post-classical Era of Yoga

Patanjali's Yoga Sutra defined yoga practice in the early part of the first millennium, and his eight-limbed path became a central aspect of the yoga systems that followed. The Yoga Sutra, however, was firmly rooted in the dualism of Samkhya philosophy and the Gita. Certain concepts and tenets from Patanjali and the early Upanishads continue unchanged or only slightly modified throughout the post-classical period. Schools such as tantra or hatha yoga, which took exception to or radically departed from many of these older tenets, expanded the practice of yoga in often radical ways.

The one thing both mainstream and new-age post-classical philosophers had in common was their rejection of Patanjali's dualistic world view. That marked the close of one era and the beginning of a new one.

For Patanjali it was purusha and the non-dualistic tradition of Advaita Vedanta called it Atman or Self. Although this Atman resides in each one of us, he (purusha may be formless, but he's still considered to be male) cannot be understood by the senses-he can't be seen, heard, smelled, touched, or tasted. Both schools understood that humans suffer when they become disconnected from this higher Self, and both believed that liberation comes when humans realise their true, transcendental Self.

A person could free himself from suffering only when he let go of his attachments to such things and realised-not with the intellect, but with the heart-that the transcendental Self resided within and that the Self was the ultimate reality. For the non-dualist in pre- and post-classical yoga, suffering began when an individual tried to make a distinction between Self and no-Self; when he failed to understand that he was a small part of something much larger than himself; when he forgot that everything he did, all that he sensed, was simply a manifestation of the transcendental Atman or purusha. A non-dualist released himself from suffering when he came to understand that his Self was not separate, but an integral part of the transcendental Self or Atman.

It's somewhat easier to see the Divine in the mundane when you take the non-dualistic view of reality, because the Divine is everywhere and in everything. When Atman or purusha is separate, how can anyone glimpse its luminous nature in everyday life? Patanjali never really answered that question, but later commentators explained that by practicing yoga (the eight-limbed path), the yogi attains the highest level of existence. At this point prakriti becomes so transparent and illuminating (sattvic) that purusha, the transcendental Self, shines through and reveals himself. The path towards true liberation lies in experiencing (not just believing) the universe as one. This combination of jnana yoga (yoga of wisdom and knowledge) and karma yoga (yoga of taking action) is similar to the ideas espoused in the Bhagavad Gita.

Tantra Yoga

Tantra emerged early in the post-classical period, around the fourth century C.E., but didn't reach its full flowering until 500 to 600 years later. This school represents a rather radical departure for yoga philosophy. In what could only have been understood as heresy, tantra rejected the Vedas as irrelevant. It refuted the notion that liberation could be attained only through rigorous asceticism and meditation, and it dismissed the Samkhyan precept that a yogi must renounce the world in order to free himself from it. Tantra also eschewed karma yoga (the path of action or service), choosing instead to focus on devotion (bhakti), most particularly worship of the Goddess.

In teaching about the causes of suffering and the path to liberation, tantra shares common ground with its ancestors. Like the non-dualistic authors of the early Upanishads, tantric yogis believed that human suffering comes from the illusion of opposites, from the mistaken notion that the Self is somehow separate from the objects it desires. Being good non-dualists, tantrikas (tantric yogis) see all possible sets of opposites, all dualities (good and evil, hot and cold, hard and soft, male and female) contained within the universal consciousness. The only way a yogi can liberate himself from suffering, according to tantra, is to unite all the opposites or dualities in his own body. Like

Patanjali, tantrikas believe in the need to have a strong, pure physical body.

Tantrika, on the other hand, celebrated the physical body, which they considered to be a sacred temple of the Divine, as a means to conquer death. The body became the vehicle for attaining liberation. In tantric yoga, the universal consciousness, which earlier philosophers called purusha, became Shiva and resided within the body. The principle of nature or creation, called prakriti in earlier yogic thought, became Shakti and lived at the base of the spine. The ultimate unity-the male energy of Shiva with the feminine principle Shakti-took place internally and led to final liberation or Samadhi. Tantrikas believed that the whole world was not an illusion, but a manifestation of the Divine and that all experience brought the practitioner closer to his or her own divinity.

The Vamamarga, or left-handed path of tantra, employed traditionally forbidden pleasures, including sexual intercourse, to achieve samadhi. After all, they reasoned, how can an individual know what to transcend if he doesn't experience it first? The more conservative, right-handed tantrikas, on the other hand, weren't quite so literal. In fact vamamarga practices horrified them.

They considered these practices dangerous, and preferred more symbolic means of uniting male and female energies. The right-handed tantrikas relied on arduous practices of asana, pranayama, mudras, and bandhas to awaken the female energy (shakti), draw it up through the body, and unite it with the male Shiva at the crown of the head. Both types of tantra respected women far more than their yogic predecessors and most of their contemporaries, and revered the feminine deity (Shakti) as the necessary, active energy that made liberation possible.

Not everything in tantra broke with yogic tradition. Before a yogi could even begin tantric practices, he had to adhere strictly to the yamas and niyamas (ethical standards and moral disciplines) and the asanas and pranayamas as outlined in Patanjali's eight-limbed path in the Yoga Sutra. From there, the adept learned to concentrate (pratyahara) on a single point (ekagraha); for a tantrika, this point was an icon of a deity. Once he mastered pratyahara, he was ready to study visualisation, which included feeling the deity's presence and summoning the sacred force of the deity in order to experience its divinity.

Similarly, tantra's use of mantras (sacred sounds) is as old as the Rig Veda, but tantrikas employed these sounds in a very different way. Each letter of the mantra (given to the student by his guru) corresponded to a place in the body and each place in the body represented a force in the universe. By chanting the mantra, the yogi could awaken the body and its corresponding universal forces. In order to practice this form of mantra meditation, the body must be pure and strong and the mind clear and alert.

Tantric yogis liked to use visual aids, such as mandalas, in their meditations. Generally made of wood, paper, or cloth, tantric mandalas were drawings of circles and geometric designs. Regardless of how simple or complex these drawings were, they always contained a seed or beeja at the center, which represented the union of the cosmos and the mind; concentric circles, which represented the various levels of existence; and a square "fence" around the circles, with open gates, to protect the sacred space. Ultimately, by meditating and visualising, the tantrika entered into the mandala and realised that the unity of all things resided in him and that there was no separation between him and the Divine.

Yoga Comes West

The American brand of yoga we love today focuses primarily on the physical poses called asanas and is thus clearly an offshoot of hatha yoga, even though jnana yoga (the path of knowledge) and the raja yoga of Patanjali's Yoga Sutra were the first to gain currency in the West. Like Indian yogis, the first Westerners to encounter yoga were more interested in-and fascinated by-methods and practices that took them out of their bodies, transcending the physical to put them in closer touch with the absolute.

Nearly 50 years before yoga landed on American shores, a group of Englishmen formed the Asiatic Society of Bengal (in Calcutta) and took it upon themselves to study all things Indian. Their research and translations included essays on the Vedas, yoga, and the poetry of Shankara (800 c.e.). Society member Sir Charles Wilkins published the first English-language translation of the Bhagavad Gita in 1785, his colleague Sir William Jones weighed in with his own translations of the Isha Upanishad and a collection of hymns from the Vedas, and Henry Thomas Colebrooke wrote essays on the Vedas and on yoga, most particularly the Samkhya Karika, Ishvara Krishna's commentary on Samkhya.

The contemplative paths of yoga also resonated with a group of American intellectuals and self-described transcendentalists that included Henry David Thoreau and Ralph Waldo Emerson and that drew inspiration from the Bhagavad Gita. Fifty years later, Madame Blavatsky, a Russian immigrant, occultist, and student of ancient India, established the Theosophical Society in New York City and in Europe. Her writings, most particularly Isis Unveiled and The Secret Doctrine, captivated her audience with the secrets of the ancient Vedas.

By 1893 Americans were sufficiently smitten by yoga exotica to embrace Swami Vivekananda, the first Indian spiritual teacher (and perhaps the first East Indian) they had ever seen. Vivekananda spoke passionately about raja yoga at the first Parliament of World Religions held that year in Chicago, and the crowd went wild. He lectured extensively for another two years before moving on to European cities and then returning to India. When he came back to the United States in 1899, he set up the New YorkVedanta Society, a still-thriving community dedicated to four branches of yoga practice: bhakti (devotion), karma (service), jnana (knowledge), and raja (the eight-limbed path of Patanjali's Yoga Sutra).

About the same time, the Germans discovered the beauty of the Sanskrit language and the mystery of the Vedas. Although several scholars of the Romantic era welcomed the rich literature of India, Max Muller, comparative religions pioneer, most influenced Vedic scholarship and helped birth the flurry of European translations of ancient Indian texts that continued throughout the nineteenth and into the twentieth century. Among the greatest of these was the work of Johann Wilhelm Hauer, who, according to Feuerstein, was the first to study the history of the Vedas. He produced a translation of Patanjali's Yoga Sutra as well. Of course the English and the Germans weren't the only Europeans to gravitate towards yoga research. Feuerstein mentions Poul Tuxen, a Dutch scholar, who wrote a history of the yoga tradition in 1911. Twenty years later, Swedish researcher Sigurd Lindquist published two books on yoga, focusing on its psychological aspects, and by the 1940s, the Frenchman Jean Filliozat had added his translations of several works, and Italian scholar Giulio Cesare Evola his own writings on tantra yoga.

Yoga asanas gained a little more prominence in America around the turn of the twentieth century when hatha yoga adherents began to look more seriously at the physical benefits of their practice. Back in India, partly in an attempt to shore up hatha yoga's sagging popularity, Paramahansa Madhavadasaji encouraged local scientists and medical doctors to explore the physiological aspects of asana practice.

One of his students, Kuvalayananda, established the first institute devoted solely to such exploration-the Kaivalyadhama Ashram and Research Institute in Pune, India. Madhavadasaji sent another of his adepts, Yogendra Mastamani, to the United States to set up the first American branch of the institute. Mastamani's connections with the Eclectic Physicians and Benedict Lust, the founder of naturopathy, gave yoga a foothold in the burgeoning holistic medicine practice of the day.

Up through the mid-1920s, Americans embraced a steady stream of Indian swamis coming to the West. But in 1924, the federal government imposed a quota on Indian immigration. No longer able to bring their gurus stateside, Americans traveled to India to find them. Paul Brunton, a former writer and editor, discovered one of yoga's greatest teachers, Ramana Maharshi, and wrote A Search in Secret India in 1934, to introduce him to the world.

J. Krishnamurti, an Indian philosopher, drew huge numbers of followers, beginning in the early 1930s and culminating at his death in 1986. For many, Krishnamurti epitomised jnana yoga, about which he so eloquently spoke, and his life and teachings influenced thousands of educators, philosophers, and laypeople. Krishnamurti was also an enthusiastic student of yoga asanas, spending many summers in Gstaad, Switzerland, with yoga master B.K.S. Iyengar and, later, with yogi T.K.V. Desikachar.

In 1947, Theos Bernard, another passionate student who studied in India for many years, wrote Hatha Yoga: The Report of a Personal Experience, one of the first guidebooks to yoga asanas. Indra Devi, after studying with yoga master T. Krishnamacharya in India, wrote how-to manuals and had scores of Americans bending and stretching to her guru's yoga. In 1950, Richard Hittleman, a spiritual disciple of Ramana Maharshi, began teaching the physical aspects of hatha yoga in New York City. By 1961, thanks to the power of television, Americans everywhere were learning a non-religious, decidedly unspiritual form of yoga exercise. The teacher was the same Hittleman, who hoped to convince these new converts that yoga meditation and philosophy could forever change their lives. His books, including The Twenty-Eight-Day Yoga Plan, sold millions of copies and put hatha yoga on the American map. Ten years later, yoga teacher Lilias Folan consummated

America's love of this gentle physical form of yoga in her PBS-TV series "Stretching with Lilias." Her openhearted, energetic manner convinced millions more that anyone could and should practice yoga. Today she has produced 11 yoga videos, which have sold more than 700,000 copies, and she continues to teach and lead workshops all over the world.

While America's World War II generation moved and stretched to the yoga of Richard and Lilias, the postwar baby boomers there and abroad yearned for a more spiritual awakening. These young college-age kids turned on and tuned in to Eastern spirituality in general and yoga principles in particular through Autobiography of a Yogi, by Paramahansa Yogananda. Although written in 1946, this introduction to the power of yoga spoke to a generation of young people in the 1960s and '70s who wanted more spiritual and transcendental experiences than they could get in their local churches or synagogues. Many of these seekers incorporated asanas into their yoga practice, but their primary goal was enlightenment, not perfect alignment in Downward-Facing Dog. Many of these same novices embraced the teachings of another bhakti yogi, Maharishi Mahesh Yogi, whose Transcendental Meditation enticed everyone from college freshmen to the Beatles, with its offer of experiences even more awesome than drug-enhanced trips.

Richard Alpert, a Harvard professor fired for his psychedelic experiments, found that a spiritual lifestyle could be even more powerful and life affirming than all his past acid-trips. He left for India in the late '60s and returned to America as Ram Dass, adept of Neem Karoli Baba. His book, Be Here Now, opened the eyes and hearts of many thousands of Western students.

Ashrams and spiritual communities burgeoned during the '60s and '70s, and while some taught aspects of yoga asana and pranayama, the other paths-bhakti, jnana, and karma yoga-prevailed.

A remarkable and eventful century in the history of Hinduism and of Yoga closed with the publication in 1999 of Eckhart Tolle's worldwide bestseller, 'The Power of Now'. Based on a powerful personal observation of ahamkara, ego, this is a straightforward manual setting out what can follow from simply remaining in the present moment -- or in yogic terms, resting the mind in theconsciousness of atman as witness. Thus presenting as simply as does Ramana Maharshi (one of the sources that Tolle incorporates, along with Ram Dass), both the essence and the first steps of Yoga, Tolle ushered in a 21st century full of the promise of the spiritual path for those who care to take it.

THE MIND AND THE THREE BODIES: THE FUNCTIONS AND INTERACTIONS

The Yogis consider than in addition to the gross physical body, there are other two vehicles used in the spiritual path. Each of these bodies consists of one or too much sheaths, each composed by different energies or elements, with which humans experience different aspects of their existence. All these interact with the mind in very determinate and specific ways. To attain liberation, the yogi aspirant must stop identifying with the sheaths and transcend them.

The Mysteries of the Mind

Yoga describes that one of the vehicles of the soul is the astral body. Using this body, human beings can operate in higher planes beyond the three dimensions. On the other hand, most are unaware of its existence, and how the astral body relates to the physical, and the effect of the mind on this body.

The physical and astronomical bodies are interconnected by a subtle channel that transports vital power. When death comes, such cord is severed and they become separate. For the duration of the dream state, the astral body becomes provisionally detached from the body, bringing about a different state of consciousness. Similar to the physical body, there are also senses of awareness in the astronomical body. When these are used, extra-sensory perceptions can arise. However, just as the physical senses often deceive us, in the same way the astronomical senses also have their limitations. Just like the Yoga practice deepens, these phenomena can emerge (siddhis psychic and physical powers). On the other words, the Yogi must be firm, and understand that this is not the purpose of the practice, and keep his efforts to attain liberation.

The science of Yoga also explains the different functions and characteristics of the mind. First, Yoga explains that all our experiences are the products of the mind and the impure senses, whether the physical or astral. For instance, once the mind is controlled, the experience of time and space is no longer present. To attain liberation, aspirants attempt to control the mind and the senses and unveil their mysteries. Through the practice of concentration, meditation, and Samadhi, one can deepen the understanding of how the mind works at each of its different levels (e.g. conscious mind, unconscious mind, superconscious mind and the higher mind). There are three stages of the mind. The first, the subconscious mind contain the impressions (samskaras) and is involved in instinctual knowledge. Second, there is the conscious mind, where the intellect resides. Finally the third, there is the higher mind, where intuition takes place. By becoming aware of the tree stages of the mind, the Yogi can slowly control the mind and guide it to the spiritual path, with the goal of transcending the illusory veil of Maya.

Just as evolution takes place in the animal kingdom, in the same way the instinct become too much intricate. The common human actions are mostly coming from the subconscious mind; there is no reflection on reaction. Thus, the first step to understand the mind is to become aware of one's actions, and to reflect before responding. A healthy subconscious mind should be under the controlled of the intellect, and not the other way around. The subconscious is also charged with emotions and even forgotten memories. Through the practice, the Yogi becomes in control of his emotion, transforming lower emotions like anger, into positive emotions like contentment.

Intuition is highly related with the internal silence. Intuition transcends reason, but does not contradict it. Intuition is experiential: to fully understand the insight shared by others, the intuitive mind should experience it empirically. All the way through Yoga, the aspirant slowly tunes into the intuitive mind.

On one occasion the Yogi has controlled and understood theses facet of the mind, the Yogi must then transcend them. Beyond these three stages of the mind lies pure consciousness, the aim of the practice. Once this state is achieved, the Yogi remains in a state of existence, knowledge and bliss absolute (sat-chid-ananda).

The Three Bodies and the Mind

The Physical Body (Stula Sharira)

This body is composed of the five elements (e.g. earth, water, air, fire and ether), that is, with atoms and molecules. With this body one experiences birth, change, decay, growth and death. It is believed that during sleep, one transcends this body. The sheath associated with this body is the Annamayakosa Kosha (Gross Physical Sheath). It is composed of food, and will come back to the food cycle after death.

The Astral Body (Sukshma Sharira)

This body is composed of 19 elements: 5 organs of action, 5 organs of knowledge, 5 pranas and 4 inner instruments. With this body, one experiences pain, pleasure and satisfaction.

There are three sheaths related to this body. The first, the Pranamaya Kosha (Vital Sheath is composed of the 5 pranas (each corresponding to a chakra, a region in the physical body) and the five organs of action. Hunger, heat thirst, and cold are experienced in this sheath. Second is the Manomayakosa Kosha (Mental Sheath) which is composed of the mind, subconscious, and the 5 organs of knowledge. In this sheath one experiences thinking, anger, depression, doubting, lust and delusion. in conclusion, there is the Vijnanamayakosa Kosha (intellectual Sheath). This third sheath is composed of the intellect (buddhi, which analyses) and the ego (ahamkara, self-assertive principle). Both discrimination and decision-making occur in this sheath.

The Causal Body (Karana Sharira)

This body is composed of karma and samskara. It is a record of all the previous actions one has performed. The causal body is composed of the Anandamayakosa Kosha (Blissful Sheath) where one experiences bliss, pleasure, calmness and peace.

CHAPTER

10

Ashtanga Yoga : Origins, Theory and Patanjali

No one knows exactly how old Ashtanga Yoga really is. Some claim that it is an ancient form of yoga dating back thousands of years. What we do know for certain is that this dynamic and physically challenging approach to yoga has been practiced in India for well over 100 years. The system of Ashtanga Yoga was first set out by Vamana Rishi in the Yoga Korunta. The knowledge of this text was passed on to Shri T Krishnamacharya in the early 1900s by his Guru, Rama Mohan Brahmachari. Krishnamacharya was a great yogi who taught yoga to BKS Iyengar (leading to Iyengar yoga), to his son Desikachar (leading to what became known as Viniyoga) and to Shri K Pattabhi Jois (the Guru of Ashtanga Yoga). Unfortunately no copies of the Yoga Korunta have survived the ravages of time. From the teachings of Krishnamacharya, Pattabhi Jois (known affectionately as Guruji) has developed the system of Ashtanga Yoga. Pattabhi Jois reached the age of 90 in 2005.

He has been teaching yoga for nearly 70 years and still undertakes a punishing teaching schedule six days a week at the Ashtanga Yoga Research Institute in Mysore, southern India (AYRE 2005). He also undertakes teaching tours in Britain, Europe and the United States. His grandson, Sharath Rangaswamy, is Assistant Director of the Institute and the most advanced Ashtanga Yoga practitioner in the world. He is expected to take over from Guruji one day.

The first westerners did not discover Ashtanga Yoga until they visited Pattabhi Jois in Mysore in the 1960s and 1970s. Ashtanga Yoga really took off in the 1990s when it gained popularity, partly because it was adopted by numerous celebrities, including Sting and Madonna. Ashtanga Yoga teachers accept the methods and teachings of Pattabhi Jois. Each posture is taught in a set sequence because each pose prepares the practitioner for the next one. Teachers who have taken the vigorous elements of Ashtanga Yoga and changed the techniques or the order of postures usually describe their classes as Power Yoga. The word Ashtanga means "eight limbs" and comes from the writings of Patanjali. He wrote the oldest and most authoritative explanation of yoga more than two thousand years ago. He set out his eight-fold path of yoga in just under 200 short verses (known as sutras) which could be memorised and passed down in an oral tradition. It is worth considering the eight limbs in more detail, as they are the basis for all yoga practice, whether Ashtanga, hatha, raja yoga or any of the other many approaches to yoga. The eight limbs are:-

Yama

This first limb deals with ethical standards and integrity. It provides guidance on how to behave while following a yogic lifestyle. There are five elements to Yama:-

Ahimsa -This means non-violence in our actions. As with all moral codes, how far you take this is an individual choice. Most people would agree that you should avoid physically attacking or hurting anyone else. But this issue becomes a little less clear when considering ideas like vegetarianism to avoid causing violence towards animals. Many yogis and most people in India – the home of yoga – are vegetarian for this reason. Some people interpret Ahimsa as a call to pacifism. In the Ashtanga yoga system, ahimsa is often interpreted as avoiding violence towards our own bodies, and instead showing care and compassion for the body. In such a physically demanding approach to yoga there is a danger of people pushing themselves too hard and forgetting the non-violence that should underlie an Ashtanga Yoga practice.

Satya - This means truthfulness. It is considered important in yoga for us to be who we really are by speaking the truth. If we delude ourselves and others we are much less likely to achieve the self-knowledge that yoga can bring. In our yoga practice we also need to be truthful about what our bodies are capable of and our motives for practicing yoga. If a student is practicing Ashtanga Yoga merely for the cosmetic benefits of a beautiful body, or because one of their favourite celebrities is an Ashtanga practitioner, then it is important for them to realise that fact. Facing the truth helps us to learn about ourselves and to choose the correct path in the future. Asteya -This Yama means non-stealing. Again there are clear implications about how we conduct our lives in terms of not taking from others what does not belong to us. On a more subtle level, we should not steal other people's time, space or peace of mind in the way we interact with them.

Brahmacharya - This Yama is usually interpreted as sexual continence and is a difficult concept for western minds. In the Indian yoga tradition sexual abstinence was expected until a student reached marrying age and was ready to become a householder. The reason for this is that sexual energy is considered to be a powerful force and should be re-directed and used for spiritual development. Nowadays in the West, brahmacharya is more widely interpreted as avoiding the unnecessary dissipation of sexual energies.

This doesn't mean no sex, but it does mean avoiding casual sexual encounters and being obsessed by sexual desire and allowing your life to be ruled by it. In the Ashtanga tradition some people consider that sexual activity with their partners is only appropriate on particular days of the month, depending on the phases of the moon.

Ȧparigraha -This Yama means non-covetousness. It is very tempting for yoga practitioners to become strongly attached to the fruits of the practice because it makes them feel so healthy and happy. Instead we should enjoy the fruits of the practice without expectation. Aparigraha also teaches us not to look jealously at people in our yoga class and covet their forward bend or back bend. People we practice with should provide inspiration and not negative thoughts or judgements.

Niyama

Patanjalis' second limb is concerned with self-discipline and spiritual observances. The five Niyamas provide guidance on how we should bring about purification of the body and mind to help advance our yoga practice. The five niyamas are:

Saucha -This means cleanliness. Yogis should keep themselves clean by washing regularly and keeping their environment clean and tidy. The mind should also be "cleaned" by controlling the input of information. There will be less benefit from doing yoga if you then go to the pub, drink large quantities of alcohol and spend time with people who put no value on spiritual development.

Samtosa -This Niyama mean contentment. We will never find true peace within ourselves through yoga if we feel constantly lacking in terms of our physical bodies or our material goods. Samtosha should lead us to a feeling of acceptance of ourselves and others and a letting go of the consumer values that are so prevalent in western society. Tapas -This refers to the creation of heat and to spiritual austerities. This Niyama is particularly relevant to the practice of Ashtanga Yoga, where a lot of heat and sweat is generated. The idea of austerities refers to the fact that it may be a difficult and challenging path to develop a regular Ashtanga Yoga practice, but out of this dedication and self discipline comes many benefits. Yoga is like an alchemy for the body, where the heat and austerities bring about a transformation in our minds and in our bodies. So Tapas is something we have to go through to make changes happen. Svadhyaya -This refers to the importance of studying the classic yoga texts and to the need for us to look deeply at ourselves. In order to transform our minds we need to train ourselves to think in a different way. Many wise yogis and sages have gone before us down a similar path, so looking at their work and reflecting upon its meaning for our own lives is an important part of yoga.

Ishwarapranidhana – This Niyama, which means surrender to God or to cosmic consciousness, can be difficult for westerners to accept. In a society where many people are agnostic or atheistic, this concept seems a little uncomfortable. But yoga is not a religion, and does not require any beliefs. So it is possible to interpret Ishwarapranidhana as having the state of mind where the motive for your actions and your yoga practice is to find your higher self, rather than satisfy some passing desire or want.

Asana

Asana, or yoga postures, is what most people in the West associate with going to a yoga class. Asana is the third limb of Patanjali's eight limbs, but in the Ashtanga Yoga tradition (and in most other hatha yoga traditions) Asana is the starting point. It would be difficult to teach people about Yama and Niyama first of all, because they would be unlikely to be receptive to the ideas or understand why they should lead their lives according to yoga's moral codes and observances. By contrast, the practice of asana leads students to develop body awareness, to treat their bodies with love and kindness and to relate to others with honesty and love. In other words, asana cultivates many of the qualities that are codified in the Yamas and Niyamas.

Pranayama

Pranayama is usually translated to mean breathing exercises, of which there are many in yoga. A more accurate and deeper translation of the word Pranayama is the control of "prana" or subtle energy in the body. According to the teachings of yoga, the physical body is sustained by an energy body known as the Pranamaya Kosha. This includes different types of Prana which help the body function in different ways. Prana flows around the body via a network of 72,000 nadis (or energy channels) that have parallels to the nervous system but exist on a subtle level. The most important elements of this energy system are the seven Chakras, or energy centres, which run from the base of the spine to the crown of the head. Linking these energy centres and running along the entire length of the spine in the subtle energy body are the three most important nadis - Sushumna Nadi, which runs straight up the middle of the spine, and Ida and Pingala nadis which also run the length of the spine and which criss-cross the chakras. Ida nadi is the energy channel for Moon energy which is soft, cool and intuitive, while Pingala nadi is the channel for Sun energy, which is energetic, hot and extrovert. When we talk of Hatha Yoga, "Ha" means Sun and "Tha" means Moon. So the purpose of all hatha yoga (Ashtanga included) is to balance these two main energies in the body - the sun and moon - to being about balance. One of the main tools for doing this is the breath, because the subtle energy, prana, can be controlled and moved with the breath. In Ashtanga Yoga the main breathing technique used is Ujjayi Pranayama.

Pratyahara

When we reach Patanjali's 5th limb, Pratyahara, the focus shifts towards developing techniques concerned with inner awareness and meditation. Pratyahara means withdrawal of the senses. The less sensory input going into the brain, the more likely it is that we will remain in tune with our yoga practice. In the Ashtanga Yoga system, students are discouraged from looking around or being distracted, and are instead encouraged to keep their minds focused on their breath and what is happening inside their bodies.

Dharana

Dharana means concentration. With less sensory input because of Pratyahara, students are more able to concentrate on their yoga practice. The Ashtanga Yoga system provides concentration points, or drishtis, on which the mind can focus to avoid distractions outside the practice.

Dhyana

The last two limbs are largely concerned with meditation and are therefore beyond the experience of most Ashtanga Yoga students, unless they have a separate meditation practice. Dhyana means the uninterrupted flow of concentration so that you are absorbed completely in whatever the mind is focused on. At this point the mind is very still and undisturbed. Dhyana is an advanced practice.

Samadhi

The eighth and final limb of Patanjali is Samadhi. This is a state of being that has been achieved by very few people apart from the great spiritual leaders down the ages. It is a state of oneness with the universe and with all beings. The person in Samadhi loses all sense of self and of ego and instead reaches a deep and profound state of peace and stillness. This is the ultimate freedom, the liberation of the Self and means that the person is a Jiva Mukti - a liberated soul no longer subject to the normal rules of life, death and (in the Indian tradition) rebirth. Although Ashtanga Yoga takes its name from Patanjali's eight limbs, there are many other yoga teachers who do not do a strong asana practice or follow the teachings of Pattabhi Jois but still call themselves followers of Ashtanga Yoga. These are people who are dedicated to studying and practicing directly from Patanajali's sutras, but they are not Ashtanga Yoga practitioners in the contemporary sense of the word. There are six series of postures in the Ashtanga Yoga system, but most people and most classes concentrate on the Primary Series (First Series).

The Primary Series is also known as Yoga Chikitsa, or Yoga Therapy, because its main purpose is to make the body healthy and strong by detoxifying and aligning it (Miele 2001).

The Primary Series comprises Surya Namaskara A & B (sun salutations) and then around 50 postures including standing poses, seated postures and a closing sequence. What sets apart Ashtanga Yoga from other approaches to yoga is the way that the demanding physical work of the Primary Series is all joined together by means of Vinyasa.

The word Vinyasa means breath and movement system. For every posture in the Primary Series there is a fixed number of breaths and movement in and out of postures. Most inhalations take place when the body is "opening" (reaching up or back) and most exhalations take place when the body is folding forward or "closing" (such as forward bends). Postures tend to be held for 5, 10 or 25 breaths. For each movement there is also a drishti or looking place so that the mind is focused and concentrated and awareness is drawn within the body. Internal muscles are also engaged by using bandhas (or energy seals). The theory of bandhas is covered in lesson two. This combination of Breath/Movement, Drishti (or looking place) and Bandha is called Tristana because is works on three levels - the body, the mind and the nervous system. Tristana is a coming together of elements which create the foundations for a correct Ashtanga Yoga practice.

When you move in and out of the Primary Series postures with a controlled breath and bandha a lot of heat is created in the body and it is usual to sweat. This heat is seen as purifying for the body and the heat also helps muscles to lengthen and joints to become more mobile. The result is a feeling of freedom and lightness in the body.

ASHTANGA YOGA – THE EIGHT LIMBS

Patanjali, the great yogi and sage who lived between 500 and 200 years BC, compiled and put into writing all the then existing knowledge of yoga in what are called 'sutras'. In this text Patanjali defines yoga as the path towards self-realisation.

Ashtanga' in Sanskrit means eight limbs or steps, and 'yoga' has many meanings of which the most important are: union and path. Yoga unites the body, mind and spirit. When we connect internally with our most profound essence we achieve the dissolving of duality and we connect with ourselves. It is this sensation of unity that allows us to feel connected. The second meaning refers to the path that leads us to this union.

Embarking on the path of Ashtanga Yoga assumes practicing the eight limbs. These are:

- Yama: moral codes
- Niyama: personal
- Asana: postures, or physical practice
- Pranayama: control of prana via the breath
- Pratyahara: retraction of the senses from external objects in order to begin looking inward.
- Dharana: mental concentration
- Dhyana: meditation
- Samadhi: contemplation or total union of the self and God.

The yamas and niyamas are regarded as the pillars, or the base, of this personal realisation but often they are impossible to achieve for a Westerner who has not received a religious or philosophical upbringing. For this reason, Sri. K Pattabhi Jois recommends beginning with the practice of asanas as a means of purifying the body and mind and to acquire mental clarity.

The yamas can be divided into:

- Ahisma (non-violence)
- Satya (truthfulness)
- Asteya (not stealing)
- Brahmacharya (sexual abstinence)

- Aparigraha (detatchment).

The niyamas refer to personal purification:

- Saucha (purification of the body)
- Santosha (contentment)
- Tapas (self-discipline)
- Swadhyaya (the study of philosophical texts)
- Ishwarapranidhana (devotion).

Asanas

In Ashtanga yoga there are 3 series of Asanas. The primary series, Yoga Chikitsa, detoxifies the physical body, aligns the vertebral column and purifies the body. The intermediate series (nadi shodhana) purifies the nervous system unblocking the energy channels and allowing the energy to flow freely through the shushumna nadi (spine) and the advanced series, Sthira Bhaga, (sub-divided into A-B-C-D) works on strength and stamina.

Nevertheless, even from the first day of practicing Ashtanga we can feel how the practice of asanas has an influence on our nervous system, on our mental strength (concentration) and on our state of consciousness. Our breathing becomes deeper, our concentration increases, and gradually we acquire a state of inner peace not previously experienced. The other five steps of Ashtanga yoga appear little by little with time. Patience is an extremely important element of yoga practice. It is more important to have initiated the process than to be more or less close to the finish, since the ambition to progress moves us further away us from the goal or from self-realisation. It could be said that the goal (if there is a one) is to be conscious of the present moment in which we live day by day. Being obsessed with progressing in the practice of asanas distances us from the essence of yoga because it causes the body to become tense. I have seen many people injure themselves because of the desire to advance too quickly. It is important that beginners especially are conscious of this. The body is slow and its rhythm must be respected.

Knowing and respecting the body, however, is more difficult than it appears. We can only know the body through transcendence of the physical and by accessing pranic energy. Only then, with humility, can we learn to respect it. For these reasons I believe that patience and humility are perhaps the most important qualities to possess on the yogic path. Pattabhi Jois always says "do your practice and all is coming". He advises that practising with consistency and perseverance will yield results in 100 per cent of cases. Indeed, everyone I have known that has commenced with the practice has told me the same: "my life has changed since I began practising Ashtanga".

THE EVOLUTION OF ASHTANGA YOGA

Ashtanga Yoga is a wonderful practice for the body and mind. It is an evolving practice that is changing and growing to suit people of all ages and abilities. At least that is its potential. The tradition and its changing nature can be a difficult thing to reconcile. This problem exists for all traditions, so understanding some of the principles at work is important. In most Ashtanga classes we begin with both the breath and with vinyasa, the movements in Salute to the Sun. Eventually we move forward learning the standing postures, usually in the standard order, and then the sitting postures, one or two Asana at a time.

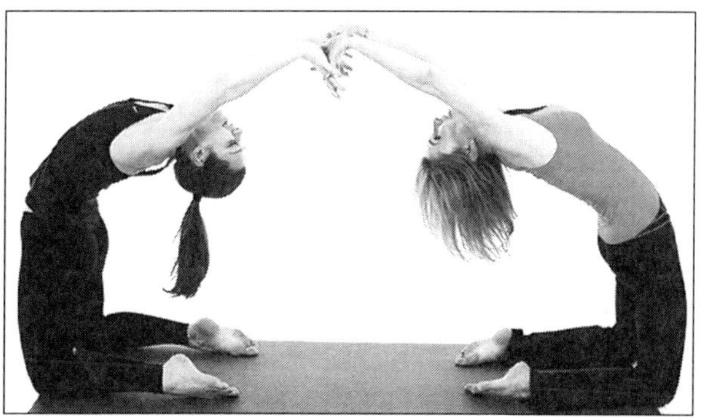

Fig. Ashtanga Yoga Asana.

At some point in this process, a student will have difficulty, physically or otherwise, and either needs to be encouraged to keep going, to focus on the standard technique, or needs to be given an alternative in order to facilitate greater ease of practice. This basic choice is true for every practice, whether it be Asana, Meditation or something else. Do you stick with the technique, tradition, or standard, or do you vary it? At what point is a variation appropriate? My thoughts on this are simple – it is not a matter of whether you vary the tradition (any tradition) but when. In terms of human evolution and holistic development, sooner or later any technique or tradition you might adhere to becomes limiting, and a lessening of your full potential.

For you to embrace a true spiritual perspective, you will need to move beyond a single method or one dimensional view. One thing we have observed, depending on when you learned Ashtanga Yoga, you will probably have a different attitude as to what the tradition actually is. Most of the teachers who learned in the 60s, 70s and 80s do not teach as strictly as those who learnt from 90s and beyond. The tradition has changed, the sequences have changed, and the style of teaching has changed. There are both good and not so good reasons for this. For example there are advantages to doing less jump backs than what is presently taught, advantages to altering some of the sequencing and changing the intensity of the practice from day to day. It is up to each of us to work out what the advantages and disadvantages are.

For me it is simply a matter of timing, of when it is appropriate to introduce either the tradition – the Intermediate Series, for example, or an alternative such as Vinyasa Krama, or Yin Yoga or meditation. That is, we would not usually introduce an alternative in the first 6 months or so of learning Ashtanga, and often longer. After the initial learning phase it is important to consider the needs of the student rather than blindly following the tradition. It is important to consider whether the standard Ashtanga is appropriate (and often it may not be) and then notice if you do not teach an alternative out of fear, rigidity or inability. We find it curious that I am one of the few traditional Ashtanga teachers to actively embrace different sequences and encourage many students to practice them - without abandoning the standard Ashtanga. We use alternative sequencing to aid and enhance the Ashtanga practice rather than to replace it entirely.

It is all about what is appropriate and practical, rather than blind faith, dogma, or just doing random stuff because we feel like it - though honestly, sometimes the latter can be really useful. Alternative sequences can enhance the Ashtanga method without altering or threatening its form and function. It is important to accept that teaching methods will vary from person to person - we are all going to teach differently with different understanding on what is appropriate. Why are the Ashtanga sequences treated as a sacred cow? It is a wonderful practice, but just Asana sequences at the end of the day. There is nothing innately spiritual, holy or sacred about them. I do think that sticking with a tradition (whatever that might be) and following the standard is truly rewarding and absolutely appropriate for most students for a period of time. Just not for everyone, and definitely not for ever.

Ashtanga Vinyasa Yoga is a relatively new system, despite some opinions to the contrary. Apart from the obvious fact that the sequences have been changed by Pattabhi Jois over the years (usually for the better in my opinion) most would agree that Prof. T. Krishnamacharya (K.P. Jois teacher) invented the system during his years at the Mysore Yoga Palace - and was influenced by the Western Gymnastic tradition, no less. I find this inspiring.

He brought together concepts from his own traditional background and made something new, vibrant and useful for people around the globe. It is only in recent times that we are seeing committed practitioners of Ashtanga Vinyasa who have been doing so for more than 20 or 30 years. The evidence for what actually works, particularly in the long term, is still emerging. What is interesting is that one of the common themes to stop practicing Ashtanga is that if it is too rigidly applied it becomes unnecessarily difficult and often injurious. Some openness towards experimentation, and the original concept of the Ashtanga Yoga Research Institute (Mysore) should still apply for all teachers and practitioners.

What Makes Ashtanga Yoga Unique

The Ashtanga Series are unique in a number of areas:

- Ashtanga Yoga is, to date, the only Yoga practice that equally develops strength and flexibility. It is interesting that all the other Asana methods on the planet, as far as I can tell, do not emphasise strength in equal measure to flexibility. There is a general bias towards flexibility. In some cases this may be appropriate (Yin Yoga for example) but in general I find this imbalanced. Why is flexibility more important than strength? Obviously it is not. One without the other is imbalanced, both physically and mentally.
- The other aspect that Ashtanga offers, that no other method does, is the emphasis on self practice. In no other method is there a greater emphasis on practice – despite criticisms towards some Ashtanga teachers, valid or not, they are all 99 per cent practicing. In addition, it takes a great deal of commitment and experience to teach Mysore style, or self practice classes, and even more commitment and experience to do it well. It is so much easier to teach led or guided classes; the latter are usually more rewarding financially also. And yet self practice is the only way to become truly meditative in your Asana practice. Why are there almost no Iyengar teachers doing self practice groups – and teaching them, not just practicing in them? The same for general Vinyasa classes, Bikram

Yoga, Anusara Yoga, Hatha Yoga, Sivananda Yoga etc. Self practice is the way forward!

- In India I have met just a few teachers of Hatha Yoga and Iyengar Yoga who conduct classes in a Self Practice format. Each was wonderfully skilled and accomplished in his own way and able to work with a diverse group of students doing seemingly random Asana independently. It takes a great deal more skill and discipline to teach self practice than it does a led class. To teach self practice really well, it also takes a lot more compassion.
- Ashtanga Yoga often seems to facilitate faster physical results than other methods. Because of the balance between flexibility and strength, and self practice 5-6 days per week, Ashtanga transforms the physical body. Keep in mind that in some cases the results can be negative - an overemphasis on physical lightness, loss of body weight and mental rigidity. Just because you are physically flexible does not make you a flexible person!
- The simple fact is that by adhering to the set sequences of Ashtanga, although more discipline is required, the results are definite. Without set sequencing, without some commitment to self practice, both the results of the body and the focus of the mind are generally limited. A key benefit of a set sequence is that it keeps you honest. You are forced to doing postures that are difficult or problematic rather than avoid them, or only doing the ones you may like or which feel good. The problem with this is that if too rigidly applied, you will then be forced into a posture that causes you injury. Avoiding difficult or problematic postures is a major flaw, particularly with styles of Yoga that don't work with set sequencing. Both beginner and advanced practitioners can fall into this trap, which leads to building up your strengths and avoiding your

weaknesses, and then leads to further imbalance, rather than less.

- Adjustments. I think one of the greatest skills most Ashtanga teachers have is communicating the practice through his or her hands. Most Ashtanga teachers give great adjustments, though some adjust too often and too forcefully. Once again, if this is too rigidly applied it can lead to injury. It is an area I think often lacking in most other systems, though part of the reason for this is led classes rather than self practice: it is easier to give adjustments in Mysore style classes because you have more time to watch and observe, rather than talking the whole way through.
- Observance of the Moon Days. Ashtanga Yoga is one of the only systems that I know that deliberately follows the cycle of the Moon, and teaches us to pay attention to this cycle and how it affects our bodies.

Some Deficiencies in the Ashtanga Method

Some observations we have made over the years show me where Ashtanga Yoga is potentially imbalanced. This is not harsh criticism of the method or the sequencing - we love Ashtanga Yoga, and still practice the Series.

They have served me well and continue to do so:

- Rajasic, Surya based Energy. The Ashtanga practice is particularly heating and upward in nature (therefore more masculine in energy) and tending to a Rajasic style practice. This is not a judgement of right and wrong - as there are both good and bad qualities to every technique, and to every person. It is futile to try to exempt Ashtanga from the human condition. For example, the Surya energy of the practice is enhanced through the linear nature of adhering to the sequences and tradition, doing right side first in most postures and focusing on drawing upward constantly with the three Bandha. I no longer find it surprising that the students who most seek to deny the Rajasic effect of the Ashtanga practice are the most trapped by this quality.

- Etymologically Surya and Rajas are synonymous, and Chandra and Tamas are synonymous. Surya is Sun, and Rajas is active. Chandra is Moon and Tamas is inactive. The combination of Sun and Moon, masculine and feminine is Sattva, or true rhythm and balance. In most modern Yoga practices, Surya and lightness are ascribed positive qualities and Tamas and heaviness are ascribed negative qualities. This merely points out the imbalance of teachers and students who focus this way. Both are important, neither is good nor bad. For this reason, some years ago, I began teaching most of my students the Moon Sequence, a combination of Yin based sequencing and gentle vinyasa. The Moon practice balances the Surya Ashtanga.
- Getting stuck on the Primary Series. In the first Ashtanga Series there is a lot of emphasis on the jumps commonly resulting in tension in the shoulders and wrists. There is a lot of emphasis on forward bends and the hamstring muscles which can aggravate many lower back conditions. This sequence does not particularly emphasise the flexibility in the shoulders, rather it develops more shoulder strength.
- It is important to balance each aspect of the body, upper and lower, between strength and flexibility. In the early years of K.P. Jois teaching the Primary Series did not have so many jumps, or so many postures. You did not jump back both sides, and many postures were linked together in groups of three and four with a Vinyasa after each set. This latter method is still useful for many students, whether beginner or more experienced.
- One of the key points of Asana practice is to open the body; which then opens the mind. Sooner or later

alternative sequencing helps to further open the practitioners' body once the set sequences of Ashtanga have been fully explored. For some students this may be halfway through Advanced A (the third series) for many students it is somewhere in the Primary Series. As most human beings cannot practice all of Primary let alone some of Intermediate, once again it is a question of when to change the sequencing. A key benefit of alternative sequencing and postures is that the practice can be tailored to individual needs, versus assuming that one or two sequences can be universally applied to all practitioners.

- Each of us has a different view of what the tradition is. So empirically it is impossible to all teach the same. So every teacher I know practices and teaches the sequencing with some kind of variation on the tradition (whether a breath, alignment, or a posture). It is just a matter of degree. Also, physically, Ashtanga Yoga does not suit everybody. It is not possible to teach it to everyone, despite what some teachers may say. If you consider the truth of that, therefore, it is a responsibility as a teacher to try to learn what you need to be able to teach anyone. Otherwise it is not Yoga, and too limited.
- For example, how do you teach someone missing one arm, or in a wheelchair? Or with schizophrenia? Although I do think the surrender and devotion to the practice (and to the teacher and tradition) is really important, it is more important to surrender to your higher purpose, the higher good, higher consciousness. Sooner or later that has to lead you from the standard approach, else you will be stuck.
- Lack of technical advice. A classical, traditional Ashtanga teacher does not teach technique classes – it is frowned upon in Mysore. Advice on how to accomplish certain postures, alignment details, and

technical advice is simply not a part of the system. Of course most teachers do offer a quiet word or two in a Mysore style class, but this is rarely done for a group. As a result many long term Ashtanga practitioners remain oblivious to many pertinent details that would help. Having said that, one advantage to a lack of technical input, is that this leads to greater devotion, surrender, and experiential learning. You can get out of your head, and just experience it for yourself without too much external stuff clouding the process. Personally I think balance between the two is optimal - time for practice without interruption, and time for clear specific instruction. A good teacher should allow for both.

- Following from point 3, here are some structural areas that often need more input.
  - Shoulder and Upper Back Sequence. My biggest structural criticism of Ashtanga and many general Hatha Yoga classes, is that most teachers do not spend much time on developing openness in the shoulders and upper back. It is just as important as any other area. For example, opening the hips and flexibility in the lower spine is emphasized a great deal more, both in Ashtanga and general Hatha classes. I often give a shoulder sequence to Ashtanga students as homework, and sometimes introduce it within the Primary Series.
  - Variations for the Hips. After teaching many Ashtangis the Moon Sequence, which has more variations for the hips, I found many students relieved and excited to add this to their repertoire. The Moon Sequence seems to have made many aspects of the Primary Series more accessible - both physically and psychologically. I have been able to introduce the Primary Series to some students who would not have done so unless they

had been introduced to the Moon Sequence first. For example many of the hip-opening postures in this sequence take pressure off the knees, relieving many knee complaints that are common with Ashtanga Yoga. For my own practice I did not need this so much when I began devising the Moon Sequence as my hips were already reasonably open. I definitely needed the energetic benefit of this sequence.

- Standing Postures and Leg Strength. Once you have worked through most of Primary, and eventually starting Intermediate and then possibly on to Advanced a few years later, despite all the possible variations you can do in the sitting postures, there are no variations that are traditionally allowed in the Ashtanga standing postures. Many Ashtangis, if not most, become strong in the upper body, some build core strength (and some do not) and few become truly strong in the legs, by comparison. The standing postures are often glossed over in daily practice, increasing the tendency for weaker legs and stronger upper bodies. This is clearly imbalanced. A regular variation on the standing sequence is useful and ideal. Although it might not be strictly 'necessary' it is so much better if you do!
- The Side Body – the area from under the armpit to the side of your hips and buttocks. There are few Ashtanga postures that work consistently with the side of the body, both for flexibility and strength – For example, some standing postures, Parighasana in Intermediate, Vasisthasana in Advanced A. Gaining better awareness, flexibility and strength in your side body is an integral part of a complete Yoga practice.

• One last aspect that Ashtanga Yoga does not utilise,

and that I have only partially used in my own teaching is the use of circular movements, either based on some kind of contemporary dance, or Chi Gung and other Chinese based practices.

The Change; Tradition vs Exploration

Ashtanga practitioners tend to be more consistent, and in order to practice 5 or 6 times per week they tend to be a little pushy also, at least in the first few years. Ashtanga attracts the character type that is more driven, and causes most students to lean in that direction. Ashtanga attracts skinnier, vata type constitutions and tends to make students change towards that constitutional type. The unfortunate fact is, the skinnier you are, the easier it is to do 95 per cent of the postures.

The important thing to consider is that some of this is good, too much is not. Accept your constitution and your experience; allow change to occur, rather trying to control the outcome. These days it is mostly accepted that Prof. T. Krishnamacharya invented the bulk of the Ashtanga sequences, borrowing many of his ideas from Western gymnastic training. I think that is a great thing, he invented something very valuable, while still adhering to many of the traditional aspects of Yoga. It is Yoga for the modern woman and man.

Since Krishnamacharya's time, Pattabhi Jois further modified, refined and adapted the sequences to his own needs and, I believe, to the particular needs of the Western students who came to learn from him. Despite denials that the Series have changed since that time, it is obvious that they have. I hope it keeps changing, because as I change and it changes, we travel and evolve side by side. As we see it, over the last 20 years, the Ashtanga tradition has become more puritanical, strict and hierarchical.

Although this may not be true in every case, across a large group of teachers and students, compared to what it was like when we first started learning, there is greater rigidity. At the other end of the spectrum, we see a great deal of variation in the Vinyasa Yoga method being taught – we would say that this is the most popular method of Yoga being taught around the planet. Given that the bulk of Vinyasa Yoga is stemming from Ashtanga Yoga, to really understand either of these completely would mean embracing both of them. There are more and more Yoga practitioners around the planet, some who see themselves as traditional, and some who do not. The traditionalists tend to be more formal, disciplined and strict, but they tend to have greater depth of experience in their particular field that the non-traditional lack.

The non-traditional tend to be more open as people, gentler and less dogmatic. If we take a peek at any of the old religions, we can see, historically the same tendency. Indeed, all societies and cultures follow this same model: the hard centre versus the expanding edge.

This is a basic truth for every method, tradition, religion and culture on the planet. For any of these to remain dynamic and stable at the same time, means embracing both polarities – every system needs to evolve else it will become stagnant, every system needs stability from which this change can flourish. It is not a question of right and wrong, it is a question of whether you can admit that wherever you sit on the spectrum, can you embrace both ends of it? Are you closer to the traditional centre, but do you deny the importance of those who change, explore and adapt? Or are you closer to the edge, finding new ways and expanding your horizons, but you find it hard to accept the strength and clarity of those closer to the centre? Embrace all of it and you embrace your full potential.

ASHTANGA YOGA – THE 'CLASSIC' YOGA

Ashtanga is the Sanskrit word for 'eight-limbed' and as written in the Yoga Sutras, the path to revealing the Universal

Self through internal purification consists of eight spiritual practices (or limbs).

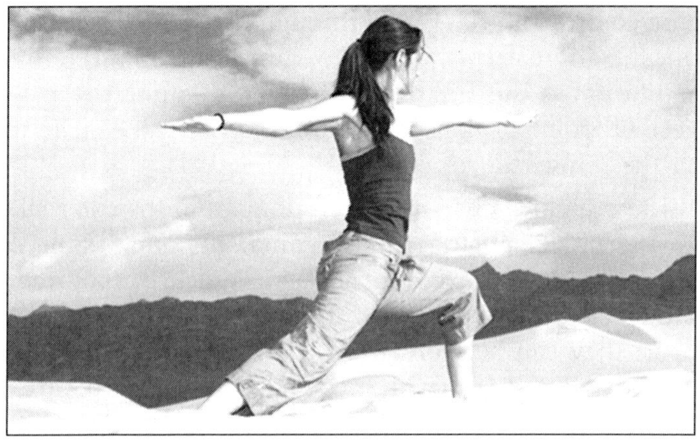

From the ashrams of India to the studio down the street, yoga has been gaining popularity in every corner of the world. As with any evolving art, different schools of practice, or subsets, emerge. Different cultures and philosophies affect yoga and an ancient art becomes contemporary and reflective of the modern way of life. Ashtanga Vinyasa yoga, or also known as Ashtanga Yoga, was popularised by K. Pattabhi Jois.

A yoga guru and practitioner from the age of 12, Jois founded the Ashtanga Yoga Research Institute in India in 1948. Ashtanga yoga was first recorded by Vamana Rishi in the ancient manuscript Yoga Korunta which also contains lists and groups of asana, original teachings, and philosophy.

The Ashtanga Yoga Composition

Ashtanga is the Sanskrit word for 'eight-limbed' and as written in the Yoga Sutras, the path to revealing the Universal Self through internal purification consists of eight spiritual practices (or limbs): yama (moral codes –consideration for others, right communication, refraining from coveting, moderation, and non-greed), niyama (self-purification and study - purity, contentment, respect to higher intelligence, and the removal of impurities), asana (alert but relaxed practice of posture), pranayama (regulated breath control), pratyahara (sense control and relaxation through inward focus), dharana (concentration - the ability to direct the mind), dhyana (meditation - the unbroken flow of thought towards an object or point of concentration), and samadhi (absorption into the Universal, or Illumination).

These eight limbs are broken down into the external and the internal cleansing limbs: yama, niyama, asana, and pranayama are the external cleansing practices that one can do to reveal the Universal Self. These practices are correctable, that is, they can be worked on until perfected. The internal cleansing limbs: pratyahara, dharana, dyhana, are not correctable. The Ashtanga yoga method can protect the practitioner's mind from dangerous corruption if the internal cleansing practices are done incorrectly. Vinyasa refers to the aligning of both movement and breath. Doing this creates a flow between different postures.

Focusing on the time it takes to inhale and exhale and then holding postures for a determined number of breaths emphasize the transition between asana and then body alignment once in the desired position. Other forms of yoga, such as hatha, focus primarily on perfect body alignment in asana and not on the breathing and movement between each posture. The vinyasa, or flow between asana, can often be seen in multiple-pose movements such as Sun Salutation (Surya Namaskara) which is a collection of 12 flowing movements. Transitioning from Plank pose to Low Plank pose and Upward-facing Dog (Urdhva Mukha Svanasana) to Downward-facing Dog (Adho Mukha Svanasana) within the Sun Salutation, for example, are vinyasa because they are flowing transitions. Ashtanga Yoga uses a specific style of breathing called ujjayi. This is a relaxed style of breathing from the diaphragm. Known for the ocean sound which resonates in the throat, inhaling and exhaling steadily in alignment with the asana creates a calming, mental focal point for concentration and relaxation. Combining vinyasa with ujjayi is said to create internal heat with causes increased circulation and sweating. This purifies the body and has led to the Western generic name 'Power Yoga' that many studios and students use today.

To complement ujjayi, Ashtanga vinyasa yoga practice incorporates bandha, or muscle locking/ contraction. This helps to focus energy in the body and is closely tied with breathing. The sustained contraction of a group of muscles also helps the practitioner hold a position and move smoothly in and out of it. The three bandha are: mula bandha (root lock, tightening muscles around the pelvis and perineum), uddiyana bandha (contraction of the muscles in the lower abdomen area, bringing the navel to the base of the spine), and jalandhara bandha (throat lock, lowering the chin while raising the sternum and bringing the gaze to the tip of the nose). Many of the asana incorporate focused gaze for concentration. Drishti in Sanskrit, these gazes help develop the internal cleansing practices of Ashtanga's eight limbs. The most popular drishti of nine is Urdhva, gazing to the sky, or upwards. It is used in the Warrior Angle pose, Balancing Half-Moon pose and Prayer pose. The remaining eight are: Angustha Madhyai (gazing to the thumb, used in Warrior I pose), Bhrumadhya (gazing to the third eye, or between the eyebrows, used in Fish pose and Upward Fold pose), Nasagrai (gazing at the tip of the nose, or at a point ten centimeters from the tip, used in the Upward-face Dog and Standing Forward Fold poses), Hastagrai (gazing to the palm, or extended hand, used in Triangle pose and Warrior II pose), Parsva (gazing to the left or right side, used in seated spinal twists), Nabhichakra (gazing to the navel used in Downward-facing Dog pose), and Padayoragrai (gazing to the toes, and used in poses like Cat-Cow).

The Ashtanga Yoga Class

An Ashtanga class is completely predefined, and rarely strays from the classic Ashtanga sequencing. Each class has four main parts: an opening sequence, one of six main series of poses, a back-bending sequence, and a finishing sequence of inverted asana. In the opening sequence, practitioners begin with Sun Salutations and several standing asana. The six series of Ashtanaga yoga form a basis of the entire system of asana. They are the Primary series (Yoga Chikitsa), Intermediate series (Nadi Shodhana), and Advanced series A, B, C, or D (Sthira Bhaga). The series allow new yoga practitioners to work through the basic asana to the very difficult ones consecutively, mastering the asana and pranayama (breathing techniques) along the way. The class will always end with savasana, or corpse pose.

Lasting an hour to two hours, a typical Ashtanga class emphasizes self-guided yoga practice. Classes can go at the practitioner's own pace and should be held daily. Many classes offered in Western yoga studios are devoted to a specific series, yet the more traditional style of teaching Ashtanga yoga is called Mysore style. Named for the city in India where Ashtanga was thought to have originated, Mysore is supervised self practice where students work to maintain internal focus while advancing to more difficult asana during practice. To stay true to the Ashtanga yoga style, many yoga studios and schools have started offering weekly or monthly Mysore classes for Ashtanga devotees who may conduct their individual classes on their mats and be properly supervised by an instructor.

THE LOGIC OF THE ASHTANGA YOGA ASANA SYSTEM

The Ashtanga Yoga asana system consists of six series, which are learned sequentially. We begin with the primary series, also known as yoga chikitsa, or yoga purification. The purpose of this series is to strengthen and purify the body in preparation for more advanced practices that follow. The primary series is an example of true genius in asana sequencing. From a physical perspective, each stage of the primary series is a vehicle to prepare for subsequent stages: Surya namaskara warm up the body, engage the bandhas and the breath, develop strength, and initiate a rhythm for the flowing practice to come. Standing postures develop stability and connection through the hips and legs into the earth. Seated postures create awareness of the hip joints and work to prepare the back for the intense work that will come in back bending.

Closing postures prepare us for post-practice reentry, resetting and stabilising the nervous activity that often surfaces during the intensity of the practice. There is an ebb and flow in the intensity of the practice.

Surya namaskara provide a gradual but quick escalation of physical activity and at the same time focus and prepare the mind and nervous system for what is to come. Standing postures further increase the intensity, which culminates in the balancing postures.

Seated postures initially seem to provide some relief but the intensity quickly ramps up again, escalating through intense forward folds and transitions which involve arm balances. We then find another seeming reprieve during reclined postures, only to arrive at the peak of the practice which comes in backbending.

Closing postures appear to put us on the downhill slope towards the end of the practice but once again we have the final burst of intensity in uttpluthi, where we have to lift ourselves up and hold for ten long breaths before finally taking rest.

Within each segment of the primary series, the sequencing of poses involves interleaved sets of poses and counterposes, which alternately strengthen and open various parts of the body.

For example, the deep forward bends of paschimattanasana, which lengthen the muscles along the back side of the body, are immediately followed by purvottanasana, which strongly engages the muscles of the back body and requires broadening and opening the front of the body. The balancing postures of utthita hasta padagusthasana require strongly engaging the deep muscles of the hip joints to create stability, and are then immediately followed by ardha baddha padmottanasana, which requires opening and external rotation of the hip joints.

Part of the rationale behind this type of pose/counterpose sequencing is that muscles will stretch more readily after they have been working and are warmed up. As a result of engaging the muscles of the hip joints, the action of working to open the hip joints that follows is more effective and safer.

Furthermore, the sequencing is structured in such a way that earlier postures in the series prepare us for the postures that come later. For example, if a practitioner is not yet able to bind in marichyasana C, then working to bring the opposite shoulder past the thigh in parsvakonasana B acts as preparation for the seated twist.

Another example is how the standing posture prasarita padottanasana A helps to prepare for bhuja pidasana through working to bring the shoulders behind the thighs in a wide-legged forward fold. There is a wealth of preparatory work in the surya namaskara – so much so that even advanced practitioners continue to find nuances within the movements of the sun salutations that carry into subsequent stages of the sequences.

It is also the case that later postures can hinder progress towards the full expression of earlier postures that have not yet been realised. For example, the core strengthening that takes place in navasana can actually make it more difficult to get into deep twists such as marichyasana C and marichyasana D, which come immediately prior to navasana.

A student who is working towards binding these seated twists, then, should not continue to navasana until they have developed the flexibility in the torso to twist deeply. Students who practice the entire primary series but choose to modify poses throughout the sequence instead of working only up to the pose that is not yet fully realised, may find that progress is slower in realising the full expressions of these poses, because the student is quite literally taking opposing actions which work against the ability to do these poses.

It is also the case that the conditioning of the body and mind which results from practicing earlier poses provides preparation for subsequent poses.

For this reason, students who attempt to force later poses when they have not correctly prepared through practice of earlier portions of the sequence, may find themselves at increased risk of injury. This is a critical point that should not be underestimated: only the guidance of an experienced teacher, who has followed this process, can guide a student through this territory.

The subtle preparatory work and its impact to the future ability to move through the sequence is opaque to the student who has yet to experience it. This is one reason why it is so important to give over control of your practice to your teacher, and to trust the process.

Many led primary classes are taught as instructional classes in which students are guided through the sequence, one pose at a time, with instruction on modifications and how to work in each pose as the sequence progresses. Unfortunately, in a led class such as this, practitioners are unable to simply flow through the sequence in accordance with the traditional vinyasa count, in which each breath and transition fits as a specific step in the sequence.

When practicing this way, students can enter a state of focused concentration, which acts as a vehicle towards meditation during the practice. When we understand how the facets described above interlace with one another to create a holistic practice, we begin to understand why the practice is traditionally taught in a group, self-practice setting. In this format, teachers can provide individual students with the unique guidance they require to work at their own levels, up to the point where it becomes counterproductive to continue. The teacher can monitor the students' progress over a long period of time and will come to know each student's degree of readiness for what comes next.

Students in this way prepare to participate in a led class which requires no instruction save the counting of the breaths, at which point the practice truly becomes one of moving meditation. When students complain about Ashtanga yoga being too rigid, too monotonous, or of being held back by a teacher, it is likely due to a misunderstanding of the method of transmission of the system. Instead, when students devote themselves to immersion within the framework of the system, trusting that incremental change will occur over time, ignoring the desire to control, and understanding the illusion of progress, they find where the real yoga happens.

CHAPTER

11

Patanjali Yoga Sutras: Principles and Practices

The Patanjali Yoga Sutras is the basic text of Yoga, one of the six great orthodox schools or systems (darshanas, views) of Indian philosophy/psychology. These six systems of thought grouped as three pairs that share metaphysical similarities are Vaisesika and Nyaya, Samkhya and Yoga, and Mimamsa and Vedanta.

The founders of these six systems are considered to be, respectively, Kanada and Gotama, Kapila and Patanjali, and Jaimini and Vyasa. The six systems can be characterised by their major emphases: particularity, distinctions, metaphysics, ontology, cosmology, and the atomic nature of reality for Vaisesika; logic and epistemology for Nyaya; exegesis of the dualism of nature (prakriti, matter and mind) and spirit (purusha, pure

This is an early, electronic version of a book chapter Braud, W. (2006). Patanjali yoga and siddhis: Their relevance to parapsychological theory and research to be published in K. R. Rao, M. Cornelissen, and J. Dalal (Eds.), Handbook of Indian psychology (in preparation). Do not cite this chapter or quote any of its contents without the written permission of the author. consciousness) for Samkhya; control of physical and mental processes through disciplined practice, with the ultimate aim of isolation, independence, or liberation (kaivalya) from the motions and changes of matter and mind for Yoga; testimony and proof, establishing the authority of the Vedas and interpreting them, especially their ritual, liturgical aspects, for Mimamsa; and the philosophy of pure consciousness and non-dualism for Vedanta.

Patanjali and Yoga Sutras

The composition date for the Patanjali Yoga Sutras is uncertain. Some place it as early as the second or third century B.C.E., a period during which the aphoristic style was especially prevalent. Some have identified the author of the Yoga Sutras with the grammarian Patanjali who wrote, in the first or second century B.C.E., a commentary (the Mahabhashya or Great Commentary) on Panini's grammar.

Others dispute these early dates, arguing on the basis of stylistic and content considerations, particularly of the fourth book or chapter of the Sutras that at least portions of the Sutras seem more appropriate to the fourth or fifth century C.E. It even has been suggested that Patanjali was a contemporary of Tirumular, author of the Tirumantiram (some time between the first and seventh century C.E.), and that Tirumular and Patanjali had a common guru, Nandi.

In the Yoga Sutras, Patanjali was a codifier and formaliser of pre-existing principles and practices. The term yoga already had appeared in early sacred writings of India (*e.g.*, in the Taittiriya and Katha Upanishads), and the practices mentioned in his Yoga Sutras no doubt had been taught and conveyed orally to a long line of spiritual aspirants.

The term yoga suggests uniting, joining, bonding, binding, linking, harnessing, yoking together; this conveys one of the two important aims of Yoga: the union of the conditioned and limited self with the true Self, of the individual soul with the Supreme Soul, the identification with purusha (pure consciousness). Curiously, the term yoga also suggests the contrary meaning of separating. For example, the commentator Bhoja described Patanjali's yoga as an effort to separate the Atman (the Reality) from the non-Atman (the apparent), and Bhoja also wrote, Yoga is separation.

Eliade (1975) pointed out that the union that is the aim of Yoga presupposes a prior severance of the bonds that join the spirit and the world... [and]... detachment from the material, emancipation with respect to the world. These dual meanings of yoga as both union and separation very closely resemble the dual meanings of the English word cleave, with meanings of both clinging, sticking, firmly adhering and splitting. The double meanings of yoga are evident in the bivalent aim of Yoga: to achieve separation, independence, isolation, liberation (from the conditioned, from prakriti) in order to achieve oneness, union (with the unconditioned, with purusha).

The term sutras literally means threads but has been generalised to refer to terse statements or aphorisms; sutras also can be taken to mean rules, principles, or formulae. Patanjali's preparation of his treatise in the form of collections of interrelated aphorisms is a carry-over from the ancient practice of oral transmission of knowledge directly from person to person (usually, from teacher to student). Brief, pithy statements allowed the material to be more easily remembered, and it also provided a mere skeletal outline, the details of which would have to be filled in by the teacher. The latter allowed more selective control of what was taught, when, and to whom, safeguarding the information from possible misunderstandings or misuse.

The filling out and interpretation of the sutras took the form of commentaries. In the case of the Yoga Sutras, important early commentaries were the Yogabhashya of Vyasa (sixth and seventh centuries), theTattvavaisaradi of Vacaspati Mishra (ninth century), the Rajamartanda of King Bhoja (eleventh century), the Yogavarttika of Vijnana Bhikshu (sixteenth century), and the Maniprabha of Sarasvati Ramananda (sixteenth century). Modern English translations of the Yoga Sutras, along with selected commentaries, can be found in Rama Prasada (1910/2003), Woods (1927), Mishra (1963), Prabhavananda and Isherwood (1969), Taimni (1975),

Vivekananda (1982), Brown (1999), and Govindan (2001). The Patanjali Yoga Sutras is a collection of 196 interrelated sutras or aphorisms, organised into four chapters or books (pada). The first chapter (samadhi pada) consists of 51 sutras that deal in a general way with special forms of attention and consciousness that are the goals of yoga. The second chapter (sadhana pada) consists of 55 sutras that describe the most important practices of this spiritual discipline. The 56 sutras of the third chapter (vibhuti pada) describe the extraordinary powers or attainments (siddhis) that can result from intense yogic practice. The fourth and final chapter (kaivalya pada), which some believe to be a later addition to the earlier three chapters, consists of 34 sutras and describes the independence and emancipation that can be the fruit of diligent yogic practice.

The Yoga Sutras treatise has been highly praised: The four books of Patanjali's Yoga Sutras, together with their ancient commentary (the Yogabhasya, which is attributed to Vyasa, the legendary poet-sage of the Mahabharata), must be reckoned among the most astounding works of philosophical prose in the literature of the world. They are remarkable not only for the subject matter, but also, and particularly, for their wonderful sobriety, clarity, succinctness, and elasticity of expression.

Nakamura (1971) has identified several characteristics of Indian thought: stress on universals, preference for the negative, minimizing individuality and specific particulars, a concept of the unity of all things, the static quality of universality, subjective comprehension of personality, primacy of the universal Self over the individual self, subservience to universals, alienation from the objective natural world, its introspective character, its metaphysical character, and its spirit of tolerance and conciliation. It is possible to detect many of these tendencies in the Patanjali Yoga Sutras.

Yoga's Aims and Practices

Yoga builds upon the metaphysical foundation of the

ancient Samkhya system, but whereas Samkhya is intellectual and theoretical, Yoga is experiential and practical. As mentioned earlier, the goal of Yoga is bivalent to achieve emancipation from conditioned matter and mind (prakriti) and to achieve oneness or union with unconditioned, pure consciousness (purusha). This bivalent aspect also is operative, more mundanely, in the practice of ordering and unifying the usually dispersed and undisciplined activities of the mind in order to eventually transcend even this more organised and controlled mental condition.

The Yoga Sutras provide step-by-step instructions for ceasing to identify with the fluctuations or modifications (thought waves, whirlpools) of the mind (citta-vritti) and for ultimately achieving complete independence and isolation from matter/mind and liberation as pure consciousness. In the course of this spiritual discipline of constant practice (tapas) and detachment (vairagya), one encounters various obstacles or hindrances (klesas, afflictions) that disturb the equilibrium of the mind: ignorance (avidva), egoism (asmita), attachment (raga), aversion (dvesa), and clinging to life (abhinivesa).

These five hindrances are the chief causes of confusion and suffering in life. Patanjali identified eight practices that help one overcome the hindrances, increase discriminative discernment, and move forward in one's psychospiritual development. These are the eight limbs (ashtanga) of yoga praxis: abstentions or restraints (yama), observances or disciplines (niyama), posture (asana), control of breath/ prana (pranayama), withdrawing sensory activity from control by external objects (pratyahara), concentration (dharana), meditation (dhyana), and absorption (samadhi). By engaging in these practices diligently and intensively, the yogin can acquire progressively greater control of body, senses, emotions, and thoughts; recognise and discriminate these limited and limiting disturbances (the seen) from one's true Self (the Seer); become capable of direct supersensory knowing; and ultimately become fully Self-realised in attaining liberation (kaivalya). At certain stages of the yogin's progressive development, various attainments or accomplishments (siddhis, powers) emerge.

Paranormal Functioning and Psi Research

Psi enquiry is used as the most general name for the scholarly approach to the study of paranormal or psychic experiences and phenomena. Other names for the discipline devoted to the formal and systematic study of paranormal functioning include psychical research, parapsychology, and psi research. The subject matter of this discipline usually is designated by the general term psi a relatively neutral technical term that suggests psychic functioning.

Psi is used to describe instances in which information or knowledge is directly acquired, or influences are directly exerted, through means other than the conventionally-recognised senses, rational inference, and motor systems. Such unorthodox, anomalous, or exceptional knowing or action can involve events that are either distant (in space and/or in time) or remote (conventionally inaccessible).

Although psychic experiences have been reported throughout history and within virtually all cultures, to many modern psychologists the very existence of psi remains controversial, and psi usually remains outside of the domain of conventional psychology. However, careful studies of psi have been undertaken for at least 120 years by scientists and scholars in professional psychical societies and organisations, institutes, and university departments in many countries. In addition, there always has been widespread interest in psi phenomena in the general public, and there has been special interest in these phenomena within the world's major religious, spiritual, mystical, and wisdom traditions, as well as within certain philosophical systems and schools of esoteric thought.

Varieties of Psi Experiences and Phenomena

Psi enquiry addresses three major types of paranormal

experiences and phenomena. The first type is receptive psi or direct knowing, in which one acquires accurate knowledge or information about events or experiences beyond the reach of the conventional senses. This form of psi has been described as extrasensory perception (ESP), psi cognition, or anomalous cognition.

Receptive psi can manifest itself astelepathy (paranormal knowledge of the mental content or experiences of others, often at a distance; a kind of direct mind-to-mind communication), clairvoyance (paranormal knowledge of some objective events, objects, or occurrences, often at a distance; a kind of mind-to-object interaction), precognition (paranormal knowledge of future events; a kind of foreknowledge or future-telling beyond what is possible through rational inference), and retrocognition (direct, paranormal knowledge of events in the past, especially of events that one might not have personally encountered, and which, therefore, are beyond the range of personal memory). Recently, the terms remote viewing and remote perception have been used to describe cases of clairvoyance, and premonition and presentiment sometimes are used to describe cases of precognition.

The second form of psi can be described as active psi or direct mental influence, but the most commonly-used terms are telekinesis (movement at a distance) and psychokinesis (PK; mind-induced movement or mind-over-matter). Recently, the term anomalous perturbation has been used to describe these instances in which physical events apparently are influenced directly and often at a distance without the use of conventional muscular or motor systems or by their extensions or tools. Psychokinetic influences may manifest as gross movements or any other changes in remotely or distantly situated objects or living systems or as more subtle changes (especially in large numbers of randomly varying events) that may not be immediately obvious to the naked eye but can be revealed through statistical analysis.

The third form of psi can be described as survival (of bodily death) or afterlife evidence. This refers to various kinds of experiences or occurrences that suggest that some form of personality, individuality, or consciousness might survive the death of the physical body. Phenomena and experiences suggestive of postmortem survival include apparitions, hauntings, poltergeist occurrences, mediumistic communications, physical mediumship phenomena, some out-of-body experiences, near-death experiences, and past-life recall and reincarnation memories.

Research and Enquiry Methods

Scientific and scholarly enquiries into psi experiences and phenomena can be carried out using four major approaches: case studies, field investigations, experimental/laboratory studies, and experiential explorations. Case studies involve the careful documentation and study of spontaneously-occurring instances of psi, with emphases on the nature of the psi experience or event, its surrounding circumstances and outcomes, the testimonies of possible witnesses, and other supporting evidence. An exemplary case study collection is the monumental two-volume work, Phantasms of the Living, published by Gurney, Myers, and Podmore in 1886, and later abridged and expanded with additional cases, respectively, by Sidgwick in 1918 and 1923. These four investigators were leaders in the professional Society for Psychical Research, founded in London in 1882 for the express purpose of carefully evaluating various claims involving paranormal phenomena.

Whereas case studies deal with experiences that usually occur non-recurrently and sporadically, field investigations are possible if paranormal phenomena tend to recur for particular individuals or at particular locations. Researchers can visit such persons or locations and conduct investigations that are more thorough, and possibly more convincing, than those that more limited case studies allow. Field investigations are common in studies of hauntings (in which possibly paranormal sights and sounds recur at particular places) and poltergeist outbreaks (possibly paranormal disturbances usually involving recurrent movements and breakages of objects; often, such outbreaks are associated with particular persons), as well as of locations such as the Catholic shrine at Lourdes, France at which unconventionalhealings are purported to take place. In addition, field studies of the efficacy of purported psychic or spiritual healers are possible. Field studies also are possible in therapeutic contexts in which paranormal content might emerge in connection with dreams or with close interactions with clients.

In experimental/laboratory studies, psi is studied under well-controlled conditions. Researchers take precautions to rule out conventional factors (confounds, artifacts) that could account for the results. Possibilities of conventional sensory knowledge, subtle intentional or unintentional cues, rational inference, chance coincidences, and fraud on the part of the research participants or of the investigator must be eliminated. If positive results are obtained under these strict and carefully-arranged conditions, and if the experiment had been thoughtfully designed and the experimental protocol had not been violated, it may be concluded with some confidence that psi actually occurred under these conditions.

In a fourth possible approach to psi enquiry, investigators may study their own paranormal experiences. This might be called an experiential approach one that involves careful introspection and reflections on one's own experiences, their circumstances and possible triggers, their accompaniments and outcomes, and their interpretations and meanings for the experiencer. Such an approach has been most strongly advocated by White (1997, 1998), especially in connection with what she describes as exceptional human experiences. This first-person approach to psi enquiry has been explored only rarely; however, it is an approach that is closely aligned with the aims and practices of Yoga.

Each of these four psi enquiry approaches has its advantages and disadvantages. The case studies approach involves experiences that are rich in meaning and life-relevance, and that sometimes serve important adaptive functions; however, the conditions under which the experiences are recorded may allow faulty observations, distorted memories, and misinterpretations. Field investigations add an element of reproducibility and fuller and more considered observations and measurements; but because the situation remains uncontrolled, troublesome confounding variables may continue to mislead investigators and contribute uncertainties to conclusions. Carefully carried out experimental/laboratory studies may effectively eliminate confounds and artifacts, but often at the cost of removing or diluting the meaningfulness and psychological salience of what is required by the test conditions. Experiential explorations allow intimate, first hand acquaintance with the studied phenomena, but this investigatory process is extremely subjective and heavily reliant upon the dispositions and skills of the individuals involved. An integral enquiry strategy that combines several methods can avail itself of the advantages of the various methods while countering their respective disadvantages.

Important Research Findings

The field investigations, and experiential explorations may provide indications, clues, and suggestions that can be followed up by more conclusive experimental/laboratory work. However, because of their more naturalistic nature, the former three methods might be able to yield unique information that even the finest laboratory studies might never be able to provide, due to the latter's intrinsic artificiality and limitations. Similar considerations apply to investigations of Yoga: Some of the more profound accompaniments and outcomes of yoga practice remain beyond the grasp of current physicalistic and rational laboratory methods.

Some of the major findings of psi enquiry are presented in this chapter. Although these have been supplemented, in some cases, by findings from the other three approaches, most of these findings derive from experimental/laboratory work. The designs of the studies generating these findings are relatively straightforward. Findings that apply to receptive psi (ESP, telepathy, remote viewing) derive from experiments in which research participants are asked to psychically perceive which of a known set of objects (*e.g.*, cards) is being displayed beyond the reach of their conventional senses (in so-calledrestricted response or forced-choice studies) or, alternatively, asked to psychically describe a randomly selected distant image, picture, geographical site, or location either by itself or as it is viewed by someone else (in so-called free response studies).

Findings that apply to active psi (psychokinesis [PK]) derive chiefly from studies in which research participants are asked to influence, mentally and at a distance, randomly varying physical systems (*e.g.*, bouncing dice, electronic random event generators based on random physical processes such as radioactive decay or thermal noise in semiconductors) or freely varying living systems (*e.g.*, changing physiological activities of other persons, changing behaviours of distant animals).

In all of these studies, precautions are taken to rule out possibilities that the results might be contaminated by subtle sensory cues (ruled out by separating the participant from the target stimuli by means of distance and/or shielding), rational inference or guessing what the target might be (ruled out by truly random selection of target events), motivated errors (ruled out by the use of blind judging techniques), chance coincidence (ruled out through appropriate statistical analyses), or normal influence (ruled out in psychokinesis experiments by choosing target systems such as radioactive decay that cannot be influenced by normal means).

For the purposes of this chapter, three types of findings are considered: (a) proof-related findings that simply demonstrate the existence of certain forms of psi, (b) process-related findings that indicate the modulating influence of particular physiological or psychological variables on the strength or likelihood of psi, and (c) process-related findings that explore variables directly or indirectly related to the principles and practices of the Patanjali Yoga Sutras.

Proof-related findings. Only a selected sample of a large number of studies that demonstrate the existence of various forms of psi can be mentioned here, and mentioned only briefly.

- A very large number of experiments have been conducted in which relatively unselected research participants were asked to guess which cards are being presented or viewed at a distant, shielded location. These are restricted-response studies in which obtained results can be statistically compared with results expected on the basis of chance alone. Meta-analyses (the application of statistical tests to the results of large bodies of comparable experiments) have indicated that participants were able to identify significantly more cards than would be expected on the basis of chance alone, effectively demonstrating the existence of psi (in the form of ESP) in these studies.
- Similar restricted-response card-guessing studies have been conducted in which the cards to be guessed were randomly selected and displayed at some future time; again, meta-analyses have indicated significant extra-chance scoring in these studies, demonstrating the existence of psi in the form of precognition.
- Extended experimental series, using the two designs mentioned above, also have been conducted with specially selected high-scoring research participants; many of these studies have yielded significant results, indicative of psi
- o Many free-response ESP studies have been conducted, in which participants in their normal, everyday state of consciousness were asked to describe

pictures that were either displayed or viewed by another person at a distant, shielded location; meta-analyses have indicated significant evidence for psi in such experiments

- Many free-response, remote viewing studies have been carried out, in which participants were asked to accurately describe distant geographical sites, buildings, and natural and human-made features that were being visited by another person; these remote viewing experiments have yielded significant evidence for psi.
- Very large numbers of experiments have been conducted in which research participants were asked to influence, mentally and at a distance, the outcomes of mechanical (*e.g.*, bouncing dice) or electronic (*e.g.*, random generators based on radioactive decay) random processes; meta-analyses have indicated the presence of psi (in the form of psychokinetic influences of inanimate target systems) in these experiments.
- Experiments have been conducted in which research participants were asked to influence, mentally and at a distance, the physiological or behavioural activities of other persons, animals, or cells; meta-analyses have revealed significant evidence for psi (in the form of psychokinetic influences on animate target systems) in such experiments. These are described as distant mental influence (DMI) or direct mental interactions with living systems (DMILS) experiments.

Process-related findings. Laboratory studies have been conducted to determine how certain physiological and psychological factors might influence the likelihood, magnitude, or accuracy of psi functioning. Such experiments not only illuminate the roles of these studied variables, but they also provide additional evidence for the existence of psi.

Here is a small sampling of investigations of factors that are relatively unrelated to Yogic principles and practices:

- There may be similarities in the processing of information acquired via subliminal perception and extrasensory perception, in terms of the psychological and brain processes involved, and there are relationships between memory functioning and ESP functioning.
- Attitudes and beliefs influence psi performance; for example, one of the classic findings in parapsychology is that persons who believe in the possibility of ESP (so-called sheep) score higher than those who disbelieve in this possibility (so-called goats) in ESP tests.
- Research participants who are less defensive tend to score higher in ESP experiments than persons who are more defensive.
- Outcomes of psi experiments depend not only upon the characteristics of the ostensible research participants but also upon those of the researchers themselves and even those of other personnel connected with the conduct of the experiments; these observed experimenter effects point to the difficulty of localising the sources of psi in any experiment.
- Psi functioning can occur and be revealed not only through conscious imagery, drawings, and verbal descriptions, but also through more unconscious physiological reactions and through changes in behaviour, perception, and memory.
- Psi functioning can be sufficiently reliable and accurate to allow the transmission of specific information and messages.

With this background on the evidence for the existence of various forms of psi, and some of the important variables that may modulate psi functioning, we can now move on to the heart of this chapter, which is a consideration of the specific ways in which the Patanjali Yoga Sutras are supported by certain psi research findings and how the principles and practices of the Yoga Sutras might enhance our understanding of psi functioning.

YAJNAVALKYA YOGA - A SIDELIGHT

In Yajnavalkya Yoga, named after the ancient sage Yajnavalkya, there are similarly eight limbs of yoga too, yet they are more encompassing, and the perspective is practice fit for living on through given methods and practices. The overall view is that proper actions help one towards greater attunements or final freedom. Yajnavalkya speaks for ten distinct yamas and alse ten niyamas where Patanjali list just five of each.

"Every little helps," perhaps. Ancient terms that head these groupings or sub-divisions of them, can have many meanings.. The sensible selection of up-to-date applications is as intended in the old book in its context, and maybe with some larger outlooks that don't negate the old ones, but go wisely along with them if that can be.

The student of Sanskrit finds up to an abundance of intertwined alternatives to the Sanskrit translations or understandings offered in Yoga Yajnavalkya and in Patanjali too. Be that as it may, the limbs of Yajnavalkya are often wider and more encompassing than those of Patanjali.

This was to make clear that Patanjali's Yoga Sutras are not the only teachings about yoga that have survived from antiquity. That point could be overlooked today.

Patanjali Yoga

A swift and deep-going mantra practice, mantrayana, may be ranked above far less effective and helpful methods. Various steps or measures from Patanjali's yoga can be added to such practice later. And gentle, safe, and pleasant yoga postures along with the mantra way are recommended.

Condensed Style

The following goes into Vivekananda's commentary on

the Yoga Sutras [in Via]. The sutras are extremely terse. The Title of the work is Patanjali's Yoga Sutras, at times translated as The Yoga Aphorisms of Patanjali. (The stress is on the second syllable, thus: 'pa-TAN-jali', with 'a' as in 'father'.)

Sutra means 'thread', literally. In this context it means thread of thought, which may also be translated into 'aphorism'. A sutra is generally a condensed statement. If condensed, it may be cryptic, or tricky. If cryptic, most persons need commentaries to derive benefits from it as intended. Traditional mentions and expert commentaries supply information that may be very helpful, and that is in fact what much of the sutra-related tradition is about.

Kingly Yoga, Raja Yoga

There are many yoga-forms, and raja-yoga is one of the demanding ones. If demanding, it may exhaust and may do havoc. If exhausting, personal interests may suffer as a result - Kingly yoga thus implies depletion of some kinds, and regular training in athletics do the same. It may not be so bad - if there is a balance between "in and out" in a "sustainable growth," broadly understood.

Some think the Yoga Sutras are the highest authority on Raja-yoga. That stand should be debated. One reason is that the thinking of Patanjali compartmentalises steps and builds that sort of thinking into a process that may not be just like that for most part. For example, novices who learn Transcendental Meditation (TM), think one sound at first, and dispense with many of the half-ritualised things of the Patanjali yoga in their training. And that is beneficial. But the second initiation (stage) of TM makes use of Patanjali topics again. Thus, the Yoga Sutras are like a menu in some respects, and one may compose a fair amount of dishes (ways) from it. ?

Sutra Renditions

Vivekananda's version is a quite free translation of the aphorisms (sutras) of Patanjali. He also supplies a running commentary, strives to avoid technicalities and tries to keep to a free and easy style of conversation.

Others have supplied other translations and commentaries, revealing differences of understanding, of interest, and of allegiances. There are many of them.

Yoga philosophy vs Samkhya-philosophy

The System of Patanjali is based on the traditional (trivial?), very old philosophical system of Samkhya. The points of difference are very few. The most important difference is that Patanjali admits the Personal God in the form of Ishvara, while old Samkhya is without a God-concept.

Gurus may warn against practising many of the things Patanjali goes into: "With few exceptions, Raja-yoga can be safely learnt only by direct contact with a teacher." It means for most people that one should let it be if unaided. Another problem is the hoary ritualism surrounding or reaching into the practice. It may be overly dogmatic in some places.

Some First Steps

Reflect on the Demanding Practice in the Beginning

For Ordinay Purpose there is inward nature and outward nature. In higher awareness than normal you have to be keen to note a difference. Quote: "Sangsara is Nirvana, and Nirvana is Sangsara". [A key dictum of Mantrayana Buddhism]. Some aphoristic expressions or teachings in the Tibetan Mahamudra School of Buddhism and Zen, can be traced back to the doctrine of the identity of the Sangsara [phenomenal world and Nirvana [realm beyond].

The study of Raja-yoga may take much time and practice. "A part of this practice is physical, but in the main it is mental. As we proceed we shall find how intimately the mind is connected with the body." THE yogi proposes to attain that fine state of perception in which he can perceive [reflect as well] different mental states.

Learn to bring Analysis to Inward States

A Yogi must avoid [extreme] austerity. [Via 585] The power of attention, when properly guided and directed towards the internal world, will analyse the mind... As for the powers of the mind, concentrated they illumine. [Via 581]

The goal of all of [Raja-yoga's] teaching is to show how to focus the mind and make it unionised through that. Thus the inward rises into attention. The later rising into broad, significant conclusions - some don't do it. [Via 582]

Raja-yoga proposes to put before humanity a practical and scientifically worked out method of reaching... its own method of investigation... A certain method must be followed... prescribed. [Via 580-81]

Vivekananda suggests, "First observe facts, then generalise, and then draw conclusions or formulate principles. [Develop] the power of observing... in order to have a real science." [Via 581]

In the study of Raja-yoga no faith or belief is necessary. Believe nothing until you find it out for yourself; that is what it teaches us. [Via 582] You may need more than ordinary staying power to stick to the training for a long time.

Practical Measures

Raja-Yoga... decrees what to do and not to do. Vivekananda: "We have therefore to take care what sort of food we eat at the beginning;... when our practice is well advanced, we need not be so careful in this respect." [Via 585]

"While the plant is growing it must be hedged round, lest it should be injured; but when it becomes a tree the hedges are taken away; it is then strong enough to withstand". [Via 585] The religion that works like some trellis, may be assisting good things. ?

Gardening knowledge can be very useful, and general knowledge is often a boon along with culinary yoga training.

Graded Steps

Raja-Yoga is divided into eight main steps and stages (above). To recap, the first three are:

- Yama - non-killing, truthfulness, non-stealing, continence, and non-receiving of gifts.
- Niyama (things to go for) - cleanliness, contentment, austerity, study, and polite and fit inward-attunement first - the greatest surrender.
- Two ways of asana (posture) - Both can be dispensed with, but preferably not: (a) Those for keeping the spine and neck steady and essentially upright during contemplation; (b) Other aiding postures for health or something else.

Pranayama

Pranayama, or control of the prana (vital energy): We get that sort of "sap" from the oxygen we breathe, from healthy food, from sun-rays and healthy life-styles. It is fine to conserve one's assets too, if that can be done, going for a much care-free life of less tear and suffering.

Vivekananda and other yogis talk of a set of three vessels tied in with the spine. They are called Ida; Pingala and Sushumna. They are not physically visible. But in certain forms of yoga there is a body of theory concerning them and other vessels called nadis. A current that is said to lie dormant, or coiled at the rear of you (near the scrotum or perineum), may be activated by intense focusing of a sort, and then the serpent power, the "Mother of eternal happiness" stings, so to speak, and in some cases rises through the middling vessel, the Sushumna - partly or completely. In the rare latter case, supersensuous illumination is had, and wisdom, self-realisation, love of God, or awakening. That is roughly how it is explained. [Via 602-03]

With pranayama training, one's face gets calmer. "I never saw a yogi with a croaking voice, " says Vivekananda. He did not meet all of them. [Via 604]

"The door of knowledge will open. No more will you need to go to books for knowledge; your own mind will have become your book, containing infinite knowledge." [Vivekananda, Via 605]. He is too pompous and grandiloquous, to be sure, granted that Vivekananda uses much book knowledge - he was studied and well versed - and not all of his key concepts are in vogue in science. "Ether" (akasha) is one of them.

Historical surveys reveal that many gurus have used different concepts, even contradictive ones. [Britannica Online, s.v. "Vedanta"]

Modern gurus contradict ancient gurus, and may also contradict other modern gurus, even themselves. Self-contradictions are not uncommon. Many such blunders and blunderbuss teachings make rational handling of the essence rather difficult to some.

However, intense focusing in an appropriate yoga way may activate "snake power" in the scrotum area or wherever it is felt at any time, and make for the relief or favourable conditions that may arise. Then "He reveals himself" and "His presence" is due to technicalities. And by the way, for the general public I make do with advocating just technical excellence in meditation and deep study along with proper carefulness in these matters. And do not be goaded by guru authority figures; that could be best for you, as goaded often shows up as misled.

Let us revert to the Sushumna theory once again. In theory, Ida, Pingala and Sushumna "are present in every animal - whatever creature has a spinal column. But the yogis claim that in ordinary beings the Sushumna is closed, its action is not evident", and "for the yogi alone, the Sushumna opens". [Via 605]. Not for the yogi alone - that is dogmatic and misleading, methinks.

You might not expect that Hindu monks teach other than celibacy as regulated in some Hindu way. But being a monk is not needed for yogic attainment, and that is the teaching of Buddha too. Awakening may be had by lay followers too.

"Avoid everyone, however great and good he may be, who asks you to believe blindly.-Beware of everything that takes away your freedom. Know that it is dangerous and avoid it by all the means in your power," says Vivekananda. [Via 608] Do question teachings that are favouring dogmatic ones, including some gurus - because sometimes their upbringing and their past rigours get the best of them - some turn bossy and wilful over serious matters; maybe greedy too.

Pratyahara

Pratyahara is "inwardmaking of the mind", making the mind turn inward. It 'shifts' that way when we fall asleep too. Through training of attentiveness one may get 'in' just by doing a few things unknown to many.

"The first lesson, then, is to sit for some time." [Via 609] As you become aware (again) that your attention has drifted (again), take it back to the practice, the training. That is an important part of progress in these waters.

I suggest: Put the mind on technical practice for many months, two or three times a day. Doing it regularly will help, because setting up a habit of this sort can help.

So, learning a good method of focusing the mind in a right sort of way for making the mind turn inward, is a key to repeated success, dealing with distractions from outside and within is another, and a third lies in regular drill. It is well to look at all of the material that goes along with a good method before you try it out, provided you are well for it.

Dharana

Keeping the mind steady in the interiorised position (or mode), perhaps by fixing the mind on some spot or a technical detail. If you can repeat a well thought mantra about thirty-five times without interruption, your mind could get a bit interiorised. What to do then, is keep the drill going with focus on practice, just that.

Deep Meditation, that is, Dhyana

Attention that is led inward (in the mind), tends to replenish the mind.

Some gurus who claim to help, get notorious in disregarding the dynamics of gliding or inside - they institute rigmarole and even "wail for God Mom" practices and other odd sorts of stuff. It can seriously disturb the fit meditative practice, and may mar the quality time you set off for training. Awareness needs training too. There is no need to undermine it or sidetrack it by shows of devotion and massa figures.

When you remain, dwell, in the pleasant states that elevated attention is wont to bring, who knows, a gate may open next? Fine progress is marked by getting freer and stronger within, happy too - it happens to many who do TM.

Samadhi

Some call it superconscious experience. It is not the end of yoga, though. It is a beginning of dangers and riches too. For example, a central concept of the major part of the ancient primer is samyana, 'together-control' - it means holding one's attention steady on something in the superconscious state. And then various distinguished attainments could be reachable. That is part of the general aim of handy yoga. Patanjali devotes much space to enumerating many of these attainments, and how to rise into them (or try for them) effectively.

No Goading

Sitting in a good posture could be beneficial. Doing gentle breathing(pranayama) can help too. It is good to let gentle breathing be followed by what normally should take the most time: the meditation training.

Helping the mind "inward" somehow comes close to falling asleep, but fit training is not for falling asleep, ideally. It may be different if you suffer from insomnia.

Practice Hints

Let good study Bring Handling Knowhow

Kurt Lewin is well known for his thought, "There is nothing as practical as a good theory." Best yoga theory can save you much pain and trouble, and you may save time to relax and cope in a good neighbourhood.

Here are three basic beginner steps or measures:

- Learn to observe and consider very simply initially. This equals unbiased observation, independent of whatever ideas and notions you may harbour through the efforts of others.
- Get handy in simple, preferably artistic and cosy enough ways by yourself.
- Study facts and consider angles and perspectives, against getting indoctrinated.

He found his innermost Self (Chandogya Upanishad)

Success in meditation and yoga rests on skills and regular, cool work, not on stiff demands and cults of belonging and so on.

A tale: A God and a demon went to learn about the Self from a sage. They studied with him for a long time. At last the sage told them, "You yourselves are the being you are seeking." Both of them thought that their bodies were the Self. The demon went back to his people quite satisfied and said, "I have learnt everything that was to be learnt: eat, drink, and be merry; we are the Self; there is nothing beyond us."

The demon never enquired any further, but was perfectly contented with the idea that he was God and that by the Self was meant the body. The god thought at first, "I, this body, am Brahman; so let me keep it strong and healthy, and well dressed, and give it all sorts of enjoyments."

But soon he found out that that could not be the meaning of the sage; there must be something else to the instruction.

So he came back and said: "Did you teach me that this body was the Self? If so, I see that all bodies die; but the Self should not die."

The sage said: "You are that." Then the god thought that the vital forces which work the body were what he meant by the Self. But after a time he found that if he ate, these vital forces remained strong, but if he starved, they became weak. The god then went back to the sage and said, "Do you mean that the vital forces are the Self?"

The sage said: "You are that." The god returned home once more, thinking that it was the mind, perhaps, that was the Self. But in a short while he saw that his thoughts were so many and diverse - now good, again bad; the mind was too changeable to be the Self. He went back to the sage and said: "I don't think that the surface mind is the Self. Did you mean that?"

"No," replied the sage; "you are that." The god went home and at last found the true Self, beyond all thought: It was Deep Mind, one and without birth or death, called endless, omniscient, and omnipotent Being - not body or the mind, but beyond them and yet manifesting through these vehicles.

Shield your Practice Too

Practice in a sensible way, preferably in a clean atmosphere: IT is natural to feel doubtful about things we do not see. [Via 587]

You may start with trying out a little thing first, and if successful, increase and repeat within sane and safe bounds.

Try to keep your body strong and healthy - clean too is neat -; body is the best we can have - you may not be able to live on earth without it - [Via 588-89]

It is quite necessary that we should find a posture in which we can remain for a long time. That posture which is the easiest should be the one chosen. [Via 586] ?

Good and skilled practice (training) is considered absolutely necessary. [Via 587]

Prana

Evolve skill from meticulous training

Your zest (or vital energy) accomplishes the activity. In the highest state of saṃadhi (it is pronounced 'sa-MA-di' with 'a' as the first vowel in 'father' and 'i' as in 'distance') we see the real thing. [Via 599] That which naturally takes a long time to accomplish can be shortened by the intensity of the action. [Via 597] And good luck. One Tends to good techniques through skills. Skill is the keyword. And by the way, prana is a complex concept, and a sampling concept.

Much Training makes Rigid or Motionless

The Vital force in every being is prana. Thought is the finest and highest manifestation of this prana. Conscious thought, again, as we see it, is not the whole of thought. There is also what we call instinct, or unconscious thought, the lowest plane of thought. [Via 593]... [R]eason is limited... The circle within which it runs is very, very limited. [Via 594]

You may remember the celebrated experiment of Sir Humphry Davy, when the laughing-gas overpowered him - how, during the lecture, he remained motionless, stupefied, and how, after that, he said that the whole universe was made up of ideas. For the time being the gross vibrations had ceased and only the subtle vibrations, which he called ideas, were present to him. [Via 594]

However, there are other explanations for the gas-drugged Davy's notions to take into account too, such as "mad persistence due to gas effecting the brain and mind".

Good theory is never Disturbed -

Pranayama has to do with breathing, but more than that too. [Via 595]. The whole scope of Raja-yoga is really to teach the control and direction of prana [subtle vital energy] in different ways. [Via 597]

Sometimes in your own body the supply of prana gravitates more or less to one part; the balance is disturbed, and when the balance of prana is disturbed, what we call disease is produced. To take away the superfluous prana, or to supply the prana that is wanting, will be to cure the disease. [This is akin to standard acupuncture theory, where what one tries to balance is labelled Ch'i (pronounced 'KI'). - TK] [Via 597]

The most obvious manifestation of prana in the human body is the motion of the lungs. If that stops, as a rule all other manifestations of force in the body will immediately stop. [Via 595]

Prana can be transmitted... but for one genuine case there are hundreds of frauds. [Via 596]

IN this universe... (each) form represents... one whirlpool in the... ocean of matter. The whirlpools are ever changing... Not one body remains the same. [Via 594]

The I Ching (Book of Changes) is based on a similar idea, that everything changes - except the structure of the I Ching.

Yogis say that... the mind can function on a still higher plane, the superconscious. When the mind has attained that state, which is called samidhi - perfect concentration - it goes beyond the limits of reason and comes face to face with facts. [Via 594]

Breathing gently can be advocated

By Yoga we can bring ourselves to the state of vibration of another plane and thus enable ourselves to see what is going on there. [Via 598]

Knowledge and control of prana is really what is meant by pranayama. [Via 592]

The Body Remembers as the Dody Does -.

Every part of the body can be filled with prana, the vital force; and when you are able to do that, you can control the whole body. That there is organismic recall is often overlooked by some.

Bibliography

Akers, Brian Dana : *The Hatha Yoga Pradipika,* Woodstock, YogaVidya, New York, 2002.

Allport, Gordon : *Pattern and Growth in Personality,* Holt, Rinehart and Winston, New York, 1961.

Anand, Margo : *The Art of Sexual Ecstasy: The Path of Sacred Sexuality for Western Lovers,* Jeremy P. Tarcher, Los Angeles, 1989.

Basu, Manoranjan : *Tantras: A General Study,* Shrimati Mira Basu, Calcutta, 1976.

Bryant, Edwin: *The Yoga Sutras of Patañjali: A New Edition, Translation, and Commentary*. New York, USA: North Point Press. 2009.

Chawdhri, L. R. : *Practicals of Mantras Tantras,* Sagar Publications, New Delhi, 1985.

De Michelis, Elizabeth: *A History of Modern Yoga*. London: Continuum. 2004.

Eliade, Mircea: *Yoga: Immortality and Freedom,* Willard Ropes Trask, Princeton, NJ: Princeton University Press, 2009.

Gordon, David : *Yoga, Brief History of an Idea,* Princeton University Press, 2011.

Haich, Elisabeth : *Sexual Energy and Yoga,* Aurora Press, New York, 1982.

Huettig, C. H. : *Principles and Methods of Adapted Physical Education and Recreation,* St. Louis, MO, Mosby, 1993.

Jaggi, O. P. : *Yogic and Tantric Medicine,* Atma Ram and Sons, Delhi, 1973.

Kaviraj, Gopinath : *Aspects of Indian Thought*, University of Burdwan, Calcutta, 1966.

Khanna, Madhu : *Yantra: The Tantric Symbol of Cosmic Unity,* Thames and Hudson, London, 1979.

Lidell, Lucy: *The Sivananda Companion to Yoga*. London: Gaia Books Limited. 1983.

Michelis, Elizabeth: *A History of Modern Yoga*. London: Continuum. 2004.

Müller, Max: *Six Systems of Indian Philosophy; Samkhya and Yoga, Naya and Vaiseshika*. Calcutta: Susil Gupta (India) Ltd. 1899.

Payne, E. : *The Shaktas: An Introduction and Comparative Study*, Calcutta, 1933.

Rele, Vasant. G. : *Mysterious Kundalini*, Taraporevala, Bombay, 1927.

Satyananda, Swami: *Asana Pranayama Mudra Bandha*. Munger: Yoga Publications Trust. 2008.

Schmidt, Toni : *The Eighty-Five Siddhas*, Stat Etnografiska Museum, Stockholm, 1958.

Sherrill, C. : *Adapted Physical Activity, Recreation and Sport: Cross Disciplinary and Lifespan*, Madison, WI, Brown and Benchmark, 1998.

Swami Sivananda Radha: *Hatha Yoga: The Hidden Language, Secrets and Metaphors*, Timeless Books, 2006.

Tattabhusan, P. H. : *Kamaratna Tantra*, Government Press, Gauhati, 1928.

Valle R. J. & King, M. : *Existential-phenomenological Alternatives for Psychology*, Oxford Univ. Press, New York, 1978.

Van Kooij, K. R. : *Worship of the Goddess According to the Kalikapurana*, E. J. Brill, Leiden, 1972.

Vasant. G. : *Mysterious Kundalini*, Taraporevala, Bombay, 1927.

Werner, Karel: *Yoga And Indian Philosophy*. Motilal Banarsidass Publ. 1998.

Whicher, Ian: *The Integrity of the Yoga Darœana: A Reconsideration of Classical Yoga*. SUNY Press. 1998.

White, David Gordon: *Yoga, Brief History of an Idea*, Princeton University Press, 2011.

White, David Gordon: *Yoga, Brief History of an Idea*, Princeton University Press, 2011.

Wiggins, Jerry : *The Five Factor Model of Personality, Theoretical Perspectives*, New York, Guilford Press, 1996.

Yogananda, Swami : *Autobiography of a Yogi*, Fellowship, Los Angeles, 1946.

Zvelebil, Kamil. V. : *The Poets of the Powers*, Rider and Co., London, 1973.

Index

❑❑❑